# Interdisciplinary Pediatric Palliative Care

Nazila Javadi-Pashaki
Zahra Taheri-Ezbarami • Somaye Pouy
Sachin Dwivedi

# Interdisciplinary Pediatric Palliative Care

Springer

Nazila Javadi-Pashaki
School of Nursing and Midwifery
Guilan University of Medical Sciences
Rasht, Iran

Zahra Taheri-Ezbarami
School of Nursing and Midwifery
Guilan University of Medical Sciences
Rasht, Iran

Somaye Pouy
School of Nursing and Midwifery
Guilan University of Medical Sciences
Rasht, Iran

Sachin Dwivedi
Clinical Instructor, College of Nursing
(Center for Excellence in Nursing
Education and Research)
All India Institute of Medical Sciences
Rishikesh, Uttarakhand, India

ISBN 978-981-97-9586-4 ISBN 978-981-97-9587-1 (eBook)
https://doi.org/10.1007/978-981-97-9587-1



This Springer imprint is published by the registered company Springer Nature Singapore Pte Ltd.
The registered company address is: 152 Beach Road, #21-01/04 Gateway East, Singapore 189721, Singapore

# Preface

Palliative care is a fundamental right of children with cancer. Palliative care can increase the satisfaction of children and their families through the management of physical and psychological symptoms. This book covers the main topics of palliative care, including definitions and principles of palliative care, pain management, communication, spiritual care, and bereavement, and it will be very useful for various fields, including nursing, medicine, and especially for personnel working in children's palliative care departments. This book will be useful for all healthcare workers, especially for nurses and physicians working in pediatric palliative care centers and oncology departments.

Rasht, Iran
Somaye Pouy

# Preface

Palliative care includes a set of services in different physical, psychological, spiritual, social, and cultural dimensions that are provided to patients with incurable disorders such as cancer. This service is a fundamental and essential need for cancer patients, and it is recognized all over the world as one of the six key pillars of cancer control. This care pays attention to the needs of patients and families through a team approach and considers the patient and family as the core of care, which leads to the creation of a desirable life and considers death as a natural process in life. The goal of palliative care is not to delay or hasten death. This care integrates psychological and spiritual aspects and provides a support system to help patients to be as active as possible until death. It also provides support to help the family adapt during the person's illness and, if necessary, during the bereavement. This care in children is completely different from the care provided in adults for reasons such as the existence of a different developmental period, different communication needs, dependence on adults, impact on the family, difficulty in decision-making, and clinical judgment. The key components of palliative care in children include physical, spiritual, and psychosocial dimensions and decision-making support in the family. In palliative care, the child and the family are considered as a whole, and integrated care is provided to them for physical, psychological, spiritual, and social problems. Palliative care is especially important for children with cancer, as a diagnosis of this disease imposes a psychological burden, emotional incompatibility, and many social problems on children and their families. Based on the experiences of developed countries, providing palliative care to cancer patients and their families can lead to better pain management and reduce the use of unnecessary treatments in the final stages of life.

In Iran, to date, palliative care has been provided sporadically in some centers, and the second center that provides palliative care for children with cancer is the 17 Shahrivar Rasht Educational and Treatment Center in Gilan Province (Northern Iran). As a result, this hospital has been selected by the Ministry of Health, Treatment, and Medical Education as a pilot center for providing palliative care to children with cancer and their families. Given the importance of palliative care for children with cancer, this book has been specifically designed to address key topics, including the basics and principles of palliative care, pain management, bereavement, spiritual care, and communication. The authors of this book hope that readers and all those interested in the fields of palliative care and pediatric cancer will benefit from it.

Rasht, Iran Nazila Javadi-Pashaki
Rasht, Iran Zahra Taheri-Ezbarami
Rasht, Iran Somaye Pouy
Rishikesh, Uttarakhand, India Sachin Dwivedi

# Acknowledgments

The authors express their gratitude to all the professors, colleagues, nurses, and doctors of the palliative care center and the oncology and hematology department of the 17-Shahrivar Educational and Treatment Center in Rasht, Northern Iran, who assisted us in writing this book.

# Contents

# 1 Principles of Palliative Care

## 1.1 Palliative Care History

The concept of palliative care dates back to the activities of Cicely Saunders in 1959. She was a nurse who worked as a research assistant at St. Joseph's Hospital in London, and at the request of the famous surgeon, Ronald Raven, she wrote a chapter titled "Management of patients at the end of life" for the six-volume book series that was published in the field of cancer. At that time, very few articles and books were published in the field of caring for dying patients, and there were no professional associations in this field [1]. In general, in the 1950s, all the attention of the treatment staff and the society was on the definitive treatment of cancer, and patients with cancer who were in the final stage of life were abandoned. Forty years later, the British government appointed Mike Richard, a breast cancer specialist, to manage the British government's cancer office, to improve services for cancer patients. He did very valuable activities in this field. Richard's activities made oncologists pay attention to symptom management in cancer patients and gradually helped to form the concept of palliative care [2]. Also, several studies were conducted by doctors, nurses, and assistants in the field of clinical and social aspects of caring for patients with cancer who were in the final stage of life, and books and articles were published. In continuation of these activities, the first modern palliative care and convalescent center was opened by Saunders and her colleagues in London under the name "St. Christopher's Convalescent Center" in 1967. This center performed various activities and provided patient care, education, and research.

The term of palliative care was first used by Dr. Balfour Mount, who worked at the Royal Victoria Hospital in Montreal, Canada, in 1974. Dr. Balfour Mount coined the term "palliative care" to describe his hospice program in Canada, and it has since been adopted worldwide. In fact, palliative care was a new model of care to meet the multiple needs of cancer patients. Management of physical problems, emotional support, and communication were considered the main elements of this care model. In palliative care, the patient and the family are considered as the unit of care, and improving the quality of life and satisfaction are its ultimate goals. To deliver this approach, an interdisciplinary team of experts was developed with the participation of all disciplines. This method of care was first used in hospital-based convalescent centers in the United Kingdom, mainly for the care of cancer patients who were in the final stages of life, and then was implemented in other convalescent centers in Europe [3].

In 1990, the first official definition of palliative care was provided by the World Health Organization, and in 1998, it also defined pallia-


N. Javadi-Pashaki et al., *Interdisciplinary Pediatric Palliative Care*,
https://doi.org/10.1007/978-981-97-9587-1_1

tive care for children. These definitions were revised in 2002, and the World Health Organization has not revised this definition. Based on the definition presented in 1990, palliative care is "providing comprehensive care for patients with incurable disorders with the aim of controlling pain and other physical, psychological, social and spiritual problems and to obtain the best quality of life for the patient and his family."

Based on the last definition presented in 2002, the World Health Organization changed the concept of palliative care from end-of-life care to care at the moment of diagnosis and introduced palliative care as an approach that aims to improve the quality of life of patients and their families (child and adult), and in order to eliminate the problems and dilemmas caused by incurable and life-threatening diseases by preventing or alleviating their suffering, early diagnosis, complete evaluation, and treatment of pain and other problems (psychological, spiritual, and physical) are carried out. This means that, for example, when cancer is diagnosed and treatment begins, a patient can access psychological counseling, nutrition services, pain management, fatigue management, and cancer rehabilitation. Such a model is also suitable for other chronic diseases. This definition emphasizes the quality of life, not the quantity, and acknowledges that death is a natural part of the life cycle. Also, the problem of "too little, too late" care in providing end-of-life care would be corrected with the new approach. This definition has several features, which include:

1. It seeks to improve the health status and prolong life; but he considers death as a natural process.
2. It neither postpones death nor accelerates it.
3. It relieves pain and other uncomfortable symptoms of the patient.
4. At the same time, attention is paid to the psychological and spiritual aspects of patient care.
5. The relevant centers provide the support system to help the patients live an active life until death [4].

Also, the relevant centers provide support to help families face the problem during the patient's illness, after his death, and during the mourning period.

The definition provided by the World Health Organization in 2002 for palliative care for children was very close to the definition of palliative care for adults and had the following characteristics:

1. Children's palliative care includes providing care in all physical, mental, and spiritual aspects of the child and the family.
2. These services start from the beginning of the diagnosis of an incurable disease for the child and continue throughout the duration of the disease and regardless of receiving treatment.
3. Health service providers should pay attention to the child's physical, psychological, and social ailments.
4. The successful provision of palliative care services requires family participation with the care and treatment team.
5. Palliative care can be provided in a hospital service center, in community health centers, and even in kindergartens.

It should be noted that some associations at the global level such as the "African Palliative Care Association" or the "Asian Hospice and Palliative Care Network" use the definition provided by the World Health Organization, while many other centers use their own definitions. All these definitions refer to how (as a specialized field or in the form of a general approach) or when (at the end of life or from the beginning of diagnosis) to provide palliative care for patients during the care process. Despite the many definitions provided by different organizations, there are common points between them, which include attention to prevention, relief of suffering, and improvement of quality of life.

We can describe palliative care as below:

- Provides relief from pain and other distressing symptoms
- Affirms life and regards dying as a normal process

- Intends neither to hasten nor postpone death
- Integrates the psychological and spiritual aspects of patient care
- Offers a support system to help patients live as actively as possible until death
- Offers a support system to help the family cope during the patient's illness and in their own bereavement
- Uses a team approach to address the needs of patients and their families, including bereavement counseling, if indicated
- Will enhance quality of life and may also positively influence the course of illness
- Is applicable early in the course of illness, in conjunction with other therapies that are intended to prolong life, such as chemotherapy or radiation therapy, and includes those investigations needed to better understand and manage distressing clinical complications [3]

## 1.2 Principles of Pediatric Palliative Care

- Respecting the dignity of the child and the family: Palliative care for the child should be done with respect for the wishes and preferences of the child and the family.
- Access to acceptable and compassionate palliative care: In addition to relieving pain and physical symptoms, doctors should provide access to measures that improve the quality of life. These measures include education, advice to the family and grief counseling, support from people of the same age, therapeutic music, providing interventions appropriate to the child's age, spiritual support for parents and siblings, and giving rest to the family. Resting the family and providing care for the sick child by caregivers other than family members will give the parents the opportunity to rest and rejuvenate, which can be scheduled for several hours to several days and alternately or if necessary.
- Caregiver support: Healthcare professionals should be supported by the palliative care team and colleagues and institutions involved in the child's death process.
- Continuous improvement of pediatric palliative care through education and research: The goal of pediatric palliative care is to add life to a child's life, not just to add more years to a child's life [3].

## 1.3 Traditional and New Perspective Regarding Palliative Care

The goal of palliative care in the traditional view is only to treat the disease. In this view, curative care and palliative care cannot be provided at the same time. Palliative care can only be provided for acute and short-term illnesses, and the patient and family do not participate in care planning. In the new view (integrated view), supportive and palliative care starts from the diagnosis of an incurable disease and is provided throughout the duration of the disease, an interdisciplinary team is responsible for the management of the disease, and the patient and his companions are fully involved in the process of the program. They participate in care, and the goal is not only treatment but also increasing the quality of life of the patient and his companions [5].

### 1.3.1 Estimating the Global Need for PPC

The estimated global total number of children in need of palliative care in 2017 is almost four million (N = 3,957,030 children). Children and adolescents aged 0–19 years comprise 7% of the total global palliative care needs. There is a slightly higher proportion of males (53.8%) than females. The majority of children in need of palliative care are in the African and the Southeast Asian regions (51.8% and 19.5%, respectively), followed by the Eastern Mediterranean region (12%), Western Pacific region (7.7%), and region of the Americas (6.2%). In contrast, the European region has only 2.8% of the total (Fig. 1.1). The African, Eastern Mediterranean, and Southeast Asian regions have the highest rates per 100,000 children (369, 156, and 103, respectively) [6] (Fig. 1.2).

The illness condition that generates the greatest need for palliative care among children is HIV/AIDS (29.6%), followed by premature birth and birth trauma (17.7%), congenital anomalies (16.2%), and injuries (16%). Cancers only account for 4.1% (Fig. 1.3). Progressive non-malignant diseases, excluding HIV/AIDS, generate the greatest need for palliative care among children in all WHO regions except Africa. Cancer generates a small proportion of the need in every region (Fig. 1.4).

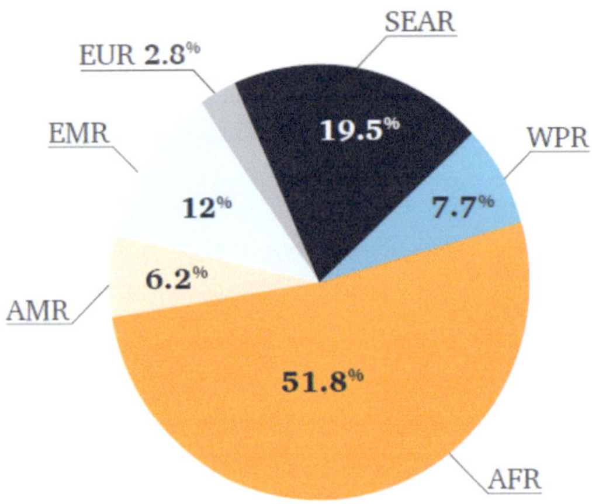


**Fig. 1.1** Worldwide need for palliative care for children by WHO region (20+ years, 2017)/N = 3,957,030 children. Source: Reprinted with permission from Connor et al. [6]

The vast majority of children (>97%) in need of palliative care live in LMICs. Almost half (48.9%) are in the lower-middle-income countries and almost one third in low-income countries (Fig. 1.5). There is an inverse relationship between the rates of children in need of palliative care and country income level. Lower-income countries have the highest ratios (Fig. 1.6).

The illness conditions that most often generate a need for palliative care in decedent and non-decedent children differ between HICs and LMICs. There are much higher numbers of non-decedent children with injuries, HIV, and congenital malformations in LMICs [6] (Figs. 1.7 and 1.8).

Maximum days of suffering were calculated for each condition and for each of the 16 symptoms occurring in these conditions in the same way as for adults, by multiplying the number of children with the possibility of having the symptom as well as the average duration of the symptom in days. For children and adolescents, the global total sum of those days of suffering adds up to over 360 million days for decedents (Fig. 1.9) and 385 million days for non-decedents (Fig. 1.10). Note that this does not consider overlap if several symptoms occurred simultaneously [6].

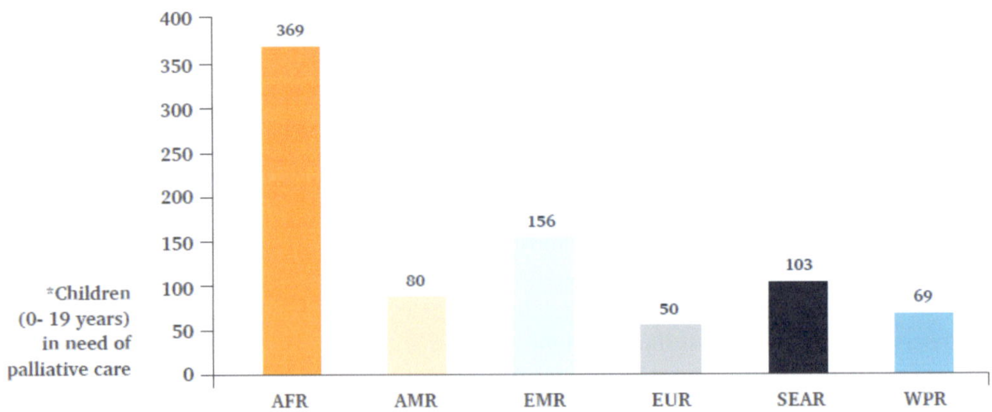


**Fig. 1.2** Worldwide need for palliative care for children per 100,000 population by WHO region (0–19 years; 2017). Source: Reprinted with permission from Connor et al. [6]

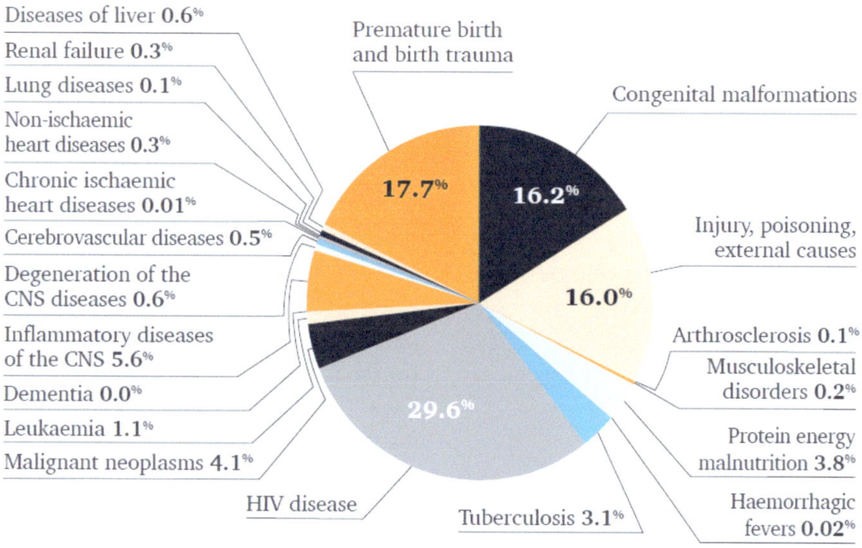


**Fig. 1.3** Worldwide need for palliative care for children by disease groups (0–19 years; 2017)/N = 3,957,030 children. Source: Reprinted with permission from Connor et al. [6]

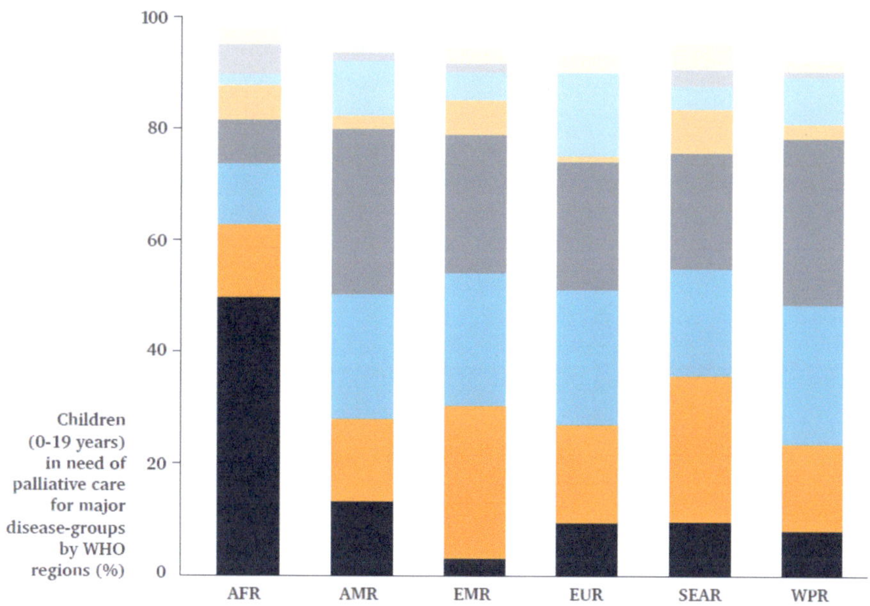


**Fig. 1.4** Worldwide need for palliative care for children (0–19 years) by WHO regions and disease categories (183 countries; 2017)/N = 183. Source: Reprinted with permission from Connor et al. [6]

## 1.4 Level of Palliative Care

Patients and their families need different levels of services in terms of their specialization. According to the estimate of the World Health Organization, nearly 80% of those in need of supportive care need only basic and non-specialized care, and only 20% of patients need specialized services. For this reason, people with appropriate expertise in the palliative care system are responsible for providing services at each level of care. In general, palliative care services can be provided at four levels, which are:

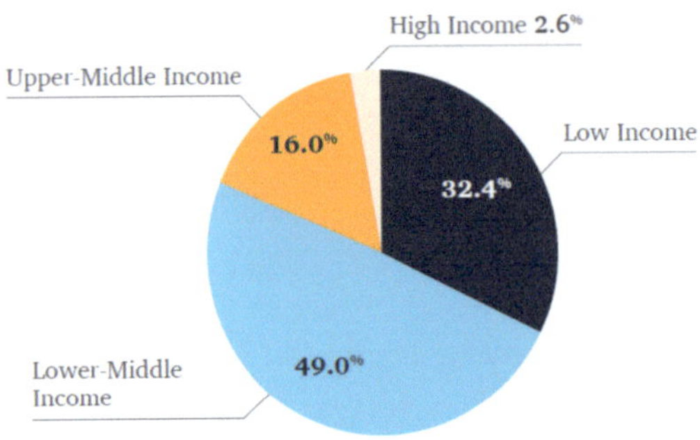


**Fig. 1.5** Worldwide need for palliative care for children (0–19 years) by income group (183 countries; 2017). Source: Reprinted with permission from Connor et al. [6]

Level zero: Providing care at the community level. Palliative care at a non-specialist level is provided by social volunteers or relatives of the patient in consultation with the doctor. Examples of these services include physiotherapy care, nutritional care, and common painkillers.

Level 1 (primary): Providing care at a more specialized level than level zero. General doctors together with the palliative care team (social volunteers or paramedics and nurses) visit and care for the patient at this level. Some actions at this level include prescribing some narcotics and managing some symptoms.

Level 2 (secondary): The specialized palliative care team including psychiatrist, oncologist, internist, and palliative medicine specialist provides services in the convalescent center or inpatient in the palliative care department if needed.

Level 3 (tertiary): The specialized team of palliative care including psychiatrist, oncologist, internist, and palliative medicine specialist provides specialized services for patients with complex problems and if surgery or hospitalization is needed in special palliative departments [7].

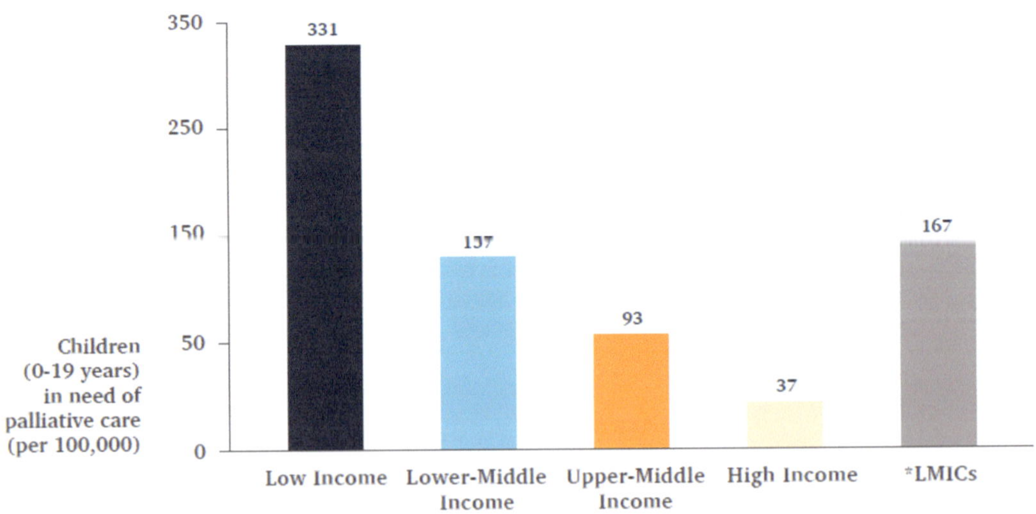


**Fig. 1.6** Worldwide need for palliative care for children per 100,000 population by World Bank income category (0–19 years; 2017). Source: Reprinted with permission from Connor et al. [6]

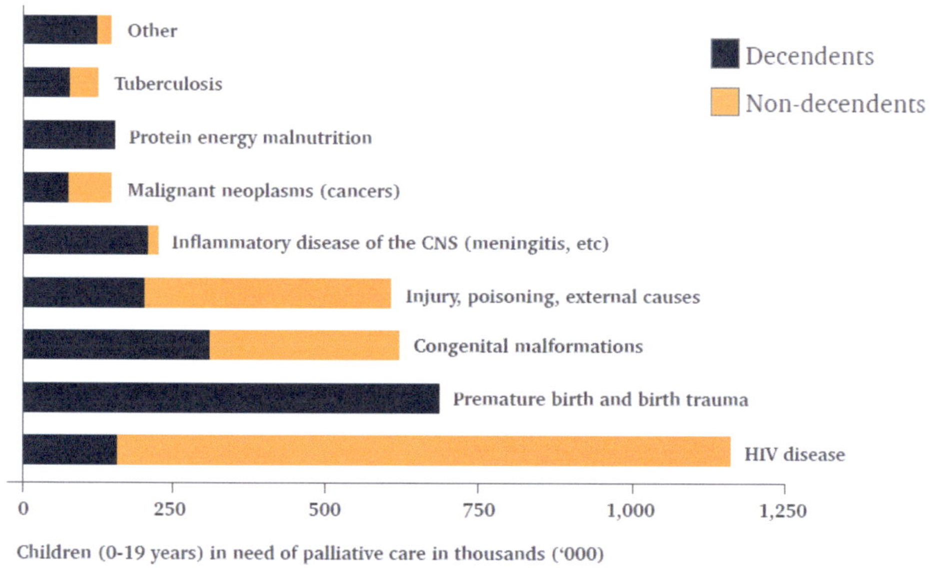


**Fig. 1.7** Worldwide need for palliative care for children (0–19 years), decedents and non-decedents, by major disease categories (2017). Source: Reprinted with permission from Connor et al. [6]

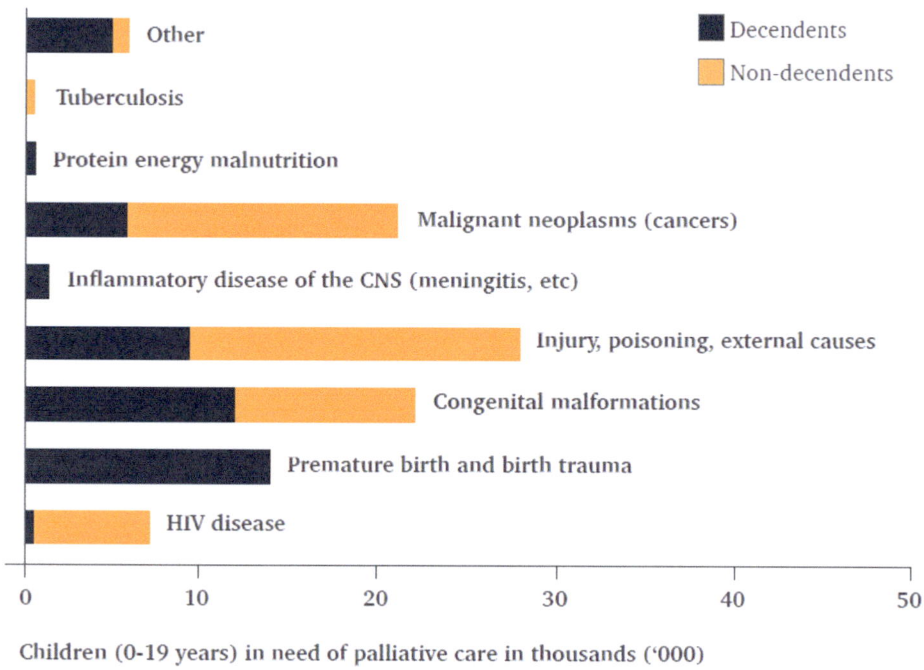


**Fig. 1.8** Worldwide need for palliative care for children (0–19 years), decedents and non-decedents, by major disease categories (2017). Source: Reprinted with permission from Connor et al. [6]

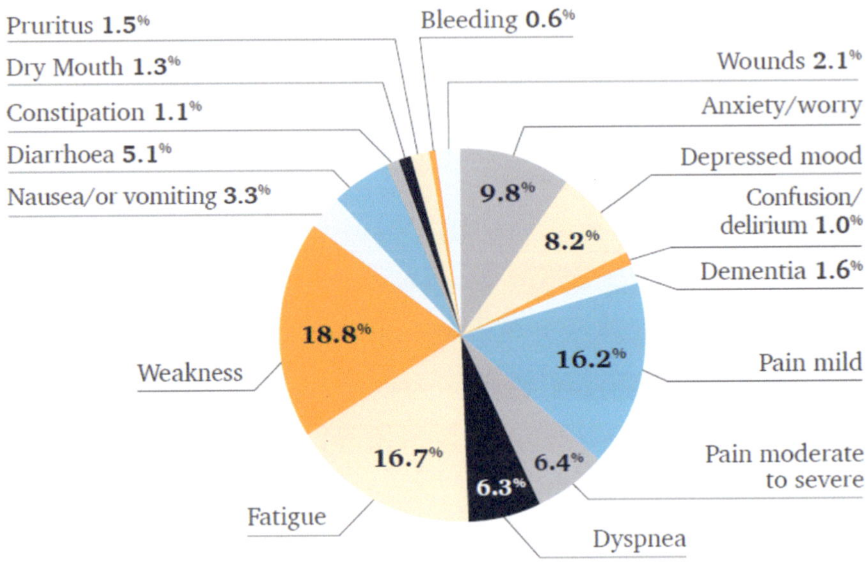


**Fig. 1.9** Percentage of days that children (0–19 years) worldwide experience serious health-related suffering for 20 health conditions (2017). Source: Reprinted with permission from Connor et al. [6]

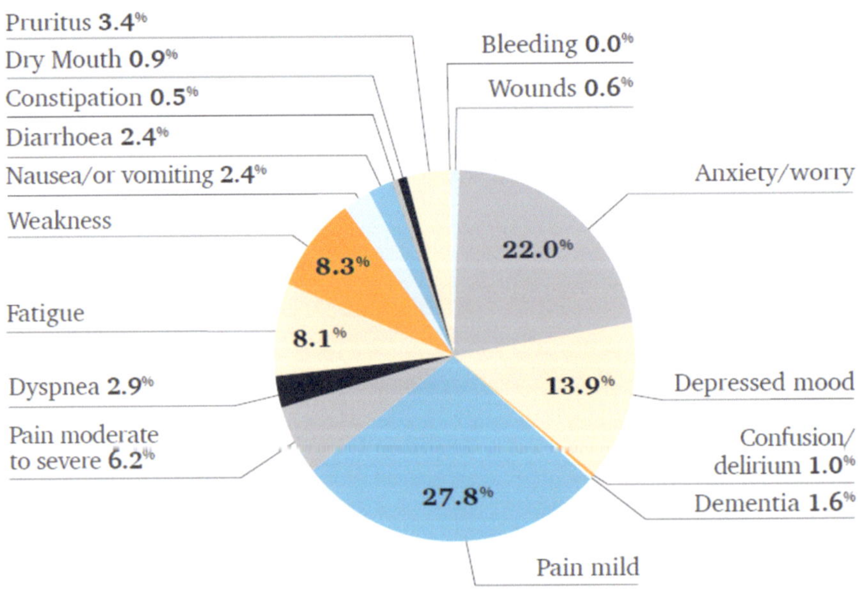


**Fig. 1.10** Percentage of days that children (0–19 years) worldwide experience serious health-related suffering by 20 illness conditions for (2017). Source: Reprinted with permission from Connor et al. [6]

## 1.5 Structure of Palliative Care

Providing palliative care services requires structures that undertake the task of providing a part of these services. Based on the place of providing palliative care, these structures should be in such a way that patients in outpatient centers, home (residence), inpatient centers, hospitals, etc. can benefit from these services without confusion and when necessary, depending on the patient's needs. In general, palliative care provision structures can be divided into two categories: hospital-based (for inpatients and outpatients) and community-based. In the following, these structures will be discussed [8].

### 1.5.1 Hospital-Based Palliative Care

Specialized hospital-based palliative care delivery structures include hospital palliative care unit (HPCU), hospital-based palliative care consultation team, outpatient) ambulatory (palliative care clinic, palliative care day service, palliative care outreach/home care service, swing beds, the integration of palliative care services with the emergency department, the integration of palliative care with the intensive care unit (ICU), and the integrated model mentioned below [9].

#### 1.5.1.1 Hospital Palliative Care Unit (HPCU)

Providing services to patients with complex needs is within the scope of duties of the palliative care department in the hospital. This department can be run in a general, specialized, or sub-specialized hospital, but it must provide services under the supervision or under the advice of a specialized support-palliative care team. These departments are created in the form of hospitals to solve some of the patient's symptoms and problems that cannot be managed at home or in some cases in convalescent centers. Relieving the patient's acute symptoms and making him stable, providing surgical services and some palliative measures, etc. are all within the scope of this department's duties. With the removal of such symptoms and problems, the patient is referred to home or convalescent centers for continued care. The most important processes and services provided by these departments can be described as follows:

- Providing inpatient services
- Providing support-palliative care services for patients with more complex needs (which the care team at home or in a convalescent center does not have the facilities to manage)
- Providing interdisciplinary care for patients
- Providing emergency services for patients with acute symptoms and needing to stabilize the clinical condition
- Providing advice to other departments of the hospital, the convalescent centers, and the home care team on a 24-hour basis
- Providing specialized training courses for doctors and nurses in theory and practice
- Providing theoretical and practical training courses for medical-nursing students [10]

#### 1.5.1.2 Hospital Palliative Care Consultation Team

This structure is considered the best structure when sufficient resources are not available to set up and run the "hospital palliative care department" or when the needs are limited. Therefore, in local hospitals that do not have an oncology department, it is useful to set up this structure at the beginning of palliative care activities. The difference between the consultation team and the palliative care unit (HPCU) is that if a patient hospitalized in one of the hospital departments needs services related to palliative care, the consultation is provided by the team members; but the team has no responsibility regarding the provision of these services and will not be involved in it. The personnel of this team include specialist doctors and nurses trained in the field of palliative care. It should be mentioned that since the task of this team is only to provide counseling, it does not require the presence of a therapist.

The most important processes and services provided by these departments include the following:

- Providing advice to the team responsible for providing primary care services.
- Follow-up of patients who have hospitalization or basic services; help and empower the patient.
- Directing the patient to receive services (taking an appointment for the patient from the clinic).
- Coordination of emergency measures with the primary service team (helping the caregivers and companions of the patient to determine whether it is really necessary to transfer the patient to the emergency room or not).
- Providing advice on palliative care at the community level: In this case, necessary measures should be taken to transfer from hospital to home (advice to home care) and vice versa [11].

#### 1.5.1.3 Outpatient (Ambulatory) Palliative Care Clinic

All over the world, outpatient clinics provide cancer patients with early access to palliative care, regardless of the healthcare system (hospital or health center) [12]. The establishment of these clinics costs very little, pays attention to the different dimensions of patients' needs, and provides access to a wide range of specialist palliative services [10]. This service is used for patients who have a good functional status and are able to go to the clinic themselves. The purpose of these clinics is to evaluate the symptoms of cancer patients and manage them by an interdisciplinary team (nurse, doctor, clergy, social worker, nutritionist, and psychologist). In these clinics, patients are visited monthly or earlier if necessary (once or twice a week) by a doctor and nurse and receive palliative care. In each visit, in addition to examining physical symptoms and problems, psychosocial issues are examined; care goals, support needs, and compatibility with the condition of the disease and according to the condition and readiness of the patient and the family are provided; and the patient is sent home after receiving the services. Sometimes at the end of each month, the palliative care nurse does the usual follow-ups by phone. In some daily clinics, in addition to therapeutic measures, there are activities such as watching TV, gardening, sewing and knitting, as well as joining creative groups that cooperate with the clinic. Therefore, social volunteers play a major role in this care model [13].

#### 1.5.1.4 Palliative Care Day Service

These services can be combined with outpatient palliative care services or counseling services and include services such as symptom management, stabilizing the patient's condition, providing counseling to the patient and family [14], preventing social isolation, leading an independent life, and reducing the responsibility of the patient's family [9].

#### 1.5.1.5 Palliative Care Outreach/Home Care Service

In this method, palliative care services are provided to patients at home by hospital-based outpatient clinic team members so that patients who do not have the ability to visit hospitals frequently, or who do not have the possibility to access well-equipped centers after discharge, benefit from the services of these services, and the team members provide services such as guidance, counseling, and home visits. Setting up these services requires very few facilities in hospitals. The most important benefits of these services are the empowerment of family caregivers [14].

#### 1.5.1.6 Swing Beds

Many hospitals do not have enough space to dedicate a separate ward for palliative care. Therefore, swing beds for palliative care patients and other patients are a suitable model for providing services in the hospital. Swing beds are actually a room that has a bed that is designed like a home environment and both patients in need of palliative care and other patients can be hospitalized. Among the benefits of this method is the effective and flexible use of the bed so that when there is no patient needing palliative care to be admitted to this bed, it can be used to admit other hospital patients. Another advantage is the possibility of distributing palliative care services throughout the hospital because patients from different departments can be admitted to this center to receive palliative care services [15].

#### 1.5.1.7 Integration of Palliative Care Services with the Emergency Department

Regardless of whether a hospital has a palliative care clinic or a palliative care consultation center, many patients in need of palliative care are often initially referred to the emergency department, where their needs are not being met. Therefore, the integration of palliative care services with hospital emergency department is required. One of the most important problems in providing palliative care in emergency departments is the lack of knowledge of nurses and doctors, lack of manpower, and legal issues [16].

#### 1.5.1.8 Integrating Palliative Care with Intensive Care (ICU)

It is a type of inpatient department that, unlike many other departments, its patients may be treated with chemotherapy or radiation therapy, although cardiopulmonary resuscitation and intubation are not performed for them. Cases admitted to the palliative intensive care unit include cancers that cause bone pain, pain caused by metastatic cancers, nerve dysfunction in the brain or spinal cord, malignant bleeding, and intestinal obstruction. Also, many patients are admitted to the intensive care unit after surgery for malignancies, and a large number are admitted to the intensive care unit mainly due to septic shock or severe sepsis or multiple organ failure. In special palliative units, radiotherapy and palliative chemotherapy are used along with other symptom control measures. This method helps in providing palliative care, controlling vital signs and managing the end of life, communicating with relatives and determining care goals, and ultimately facilitating decision-making and the possibility of choosing pre-death care for patients [17].

#### 1.5.1.9 Integrated Pattern

In this method, instead of establishing a specific clinic or training a specific group of personnel, the main focus is on teaching the principles of palliative care to all healthcare providers in a center, which leads to improved quality of life and patient and family satisfaction [18].

### 1.5.2 Community-Based Palliative Care

Community-based palliative care programs provide all care facilities such as face-to-face physician visits, specialized nursing care, equipment, supplies, and telephone support for patients at home or in a nursing home. These programs are different from regular home care programs, because in convalescent centers, more specialized care at the end of life is provided by specialist and multidisciplinary palliative care teams. In the following, the most important community-based palliative care structures are explained [10].

#### 1.5.2.1 Palliative Care in a Hospice Center

Hospice centers are places that provide high-quality spiritual, psychological, social, and physical services for patients who are at the end of their lives. In these centers, services are provided by an interdisciplinary team consisting of nurses, assistants, doctors, and spiritual caregivers. These centers provide the following services:

- Providing inpatient services for patients in an environment similar to home
- Coordinating the support and palliative care program of the patients in such a way that the patient is transferred to the hospital at the appropriate time or, in the cases of the patient's request, the necessary coordination is done with the community care team for the patient's return to his home
- Providing physical, spiritual, psychological, and social care services at a specialized and multidisciplinary level
- Providing education and training of human resources specialized in the field of supportive and palliative care
- Providing home care services (explained below)
- Bereavement care (care after the death of the patient for his family and caregivers)

Studies have shown that hospice centers lead to an increase in the quality of life, an increase in the quality of symptom management at the end of life, an increase in patient and family satisfaction with care, a reduction in invasive measures in end-of-life care, a reduction in post-traumatic stress and long-term bereavement in families. Obstacles to the universal provision of palliative care include the inability to accurately predict non-cancer diagnoses and the need to forego expensive but often beneficial treatments (radiotherapy, palliative chemotherapy, blood transfusions) due to high costs [10].

#### 1.5.2.2 Palliative Care at Home

Home care is one of the cares at the community level, the aim of which is to reduce hospital admissions as much as possible. If the needs of the patients are not complicated, it is possible to provide services at home, which is also the request of many patients. Palliative care at home includes services such as primary care; nursing care; social care; drug delivery; answering questions and providing advice.

Palliative care at home reduces hospitalization costs; reduces hospital visits and readmissions; increases patient and family satisfaction; preserves patient privacy; increases patient comfort, especially at the end of life, and family participation in providing care; and increases community awareness. Among the challenges of providing home-based palliative care in Iran are the problems related to the transfer of palliative care services from the hospital to the home due to reasons such as lack of insurance coverage, inappropriate time of transfer, and insufficient knowledge of personnel. During this process, planning for continuity of care for cancer patients is critical. Also, other obstacles include the lack of palliative care instructions at home, support for the families of cancer patients and the specialization of nurses for palliative care at home and their training, and lack of full coverage and 24-hour services to patients [10].

#### 1.5.2.3 Day Clinic

This structure provides palliative care to patients who are at home or in nursing homes. Like convalescent centers, the important distinguishing feature of this structure is a holistic view and attention to various aspects of patients' needs. In this regard, various activities including physiotherapy, occupational therapy, music and art therapy, meeting other people with the same condition as patients and establishing a friendly relationship with them in a non-clinical environment, etc. are considered in improving the condition of patients. In this situation, the patient stays at home and visits the daily clinic when necessary (usually once or twice a week) to receive palliative care. Another advantage of such centers is the low cost of its establishment. It also provides the possibility of short-term caregiving for patients' families. In some countries, the most common way of providing services in these centers is that patients are transferred to the center on certain days by a system provided by the center itself and usually managed by volunteers, and after receiving services with the same system, they are returned home. Therefore, the important issue that is raised is to think of measures that facilitate the possibility of travel for patients; otherwise, this can be very difficult for patients [10].

## 1.6 Palliative Care Models

Around the world, various models have been designed and implemented to provide palliative care services to children with cancer. It should be noted that none of these models is superior to each other and the choice of model depends on the needs, preferences, and facilities of each institution [19]. In the following, seven global models of palliative care for children with cancer are introduced.

### 1.6.1 A Three-Tier Palliative Care Model for Children

This model was presented in 2016 to provide services to children with cancer by Kaye et al. in America. This model consists of three floors. In the first floor (specialized palliative care), a team of palliative care specialists manages the physical symptoms and psychosocial needs of the child and family. In this category, the focus is on education, policy, and resource provision for providing palliative care services. In the second floor (consultation-communication), services are provided to certain groups (such as children with cancer who need surgery or children at the end of life), and referrals are made if necessary. In the third floor, the primary members of the oncology team provide counseling services based on the needs of the child and family and refer them if they need to manage complex physical or psychosocial symptoms. The initial members of the oncology team working on this floor include all pediatric oncologists, oncology nurses, and oncology interns who have received basic training in palliative care [20].

### 1.6.2 Floating Clinic

This model is implemented in Boston Children's Hospital, USA. The members of this clinic include a pediatric advanced care team (PACT), which includes six pediatric specialists, two assistants, and two nurses, and it is known as the "floating unit." The team working in floating clinic, visit the child and the family throughout the hospitalization, outpatient chemotherapy visits, bone marrow transplant and discharge, and provides counseling and support services, and also educates and follows up after discharge. In this model, members of the palliative care team meet and provide counseling services when the child and family come for an oncology visit. The results of this model have shown that it has led to the reduction of unnecessary patient visits. In this model, two nurses trained in pediatric palliative care provide the outpatient services needed by children with cancer [6].

### 1.6.3 Disease-Specific Embedded Model

In this model, which is used in the United States, a team of pediatric palliative care physicians and nurses is present in a clinic focused on disease management, such as a leukemia clinic, neuro-oncology clinic, or solid tumor clinic, along with members of the treatment staff of these clinics. Providing services based on this model leads to better acceptance of treatment and care team members and more children's access to palliative care [21].

### 1.6.4 Trigger-Based Clinic Embedded in the Oncology Space

This model is used in one of the hospitals in San Diego (USA) and is located inside the oncology clinic. The members of this clinic include a pediatric palliative care physician, a pediatric palliative care nurse, a home care assistant, and a home care nurse who work full time. In this clinic, the goal is to focus on the disease and referral of the child [21]. Therefore, if a child meets one of the referral criteria (including patients undergoing bone marrow transplantation, cancer recurrence, or, at the time of diagnosis, metastatic cancers), they will be referred to the relevant specialist. These patients are referred to a palliative care specialist based on their needs. Also, palliative care team members in this model perform actions such as coordination of care or coordination with convalescent centers. Also, the oncologist, the general doctor and the palliative care team members of the clinic introduce the family and receive advice from them if needed [14].

### 1.6.5 Consultation-Based Clinic Using Oncology Clinic Space (Embedded)

In this model, a palliative care clinic located in the Hematology and Oncology Center at Children's Hospital of Atlanta serves children with cancer under the leadership of a physician. The clinic serves as the outpatient arm of the advanced care team. PACT provides inpatient counseling services in the field of palliative care for children with cancer and includes four doctors, three palliative care specialist nurses, and one assistant and provides counseling services 2 days a week. These consulting services can be provided separately or simultaneously with the visit of the oncology team. Consultation services are also provided over the phone [19].

### 1.6.6 Telehealth Clinic

In order to facilitate the access of children with cancer and their families to palliative care services in rural and disadvantaged areas, this clinic was opened in America. In this model, palliative care team members are based in the hospital and dedicate 1 day a week to online visits or home visits (according to families' requests). The day of the visit is determined in a flexible manner during prior coordination with the families. All visits are done by an interdisciplinary team, and families have the right to choose a caregiver (such as a convalescent nurse or pediatrician) in the final stage of their child's life. Although, in this model, it is difficult to coordinate with different members of the interdisciplinary team and families for visits, it has many benefits such as reducing unnecessary visits, providing comfortable care at home, and increasing cooperation between community members [19].

### 1.6.7 Hub-Spoke Model of Palliative Care

This model was designed by Khanali et al. in 2016 in Iran. This model includes a palliative care clinic in two formats based on the hospital (under the title of hub) or independently (under the title of spoke), which is considered as the main center for providing services. Through communication with other centers, including general clinics, home care centers, general hospitals, and specialized children's hospitals, the clinic facilitates access to services and coordinates and manages the provision of services in the aforementioned centers.

In a hospital-based format, the main and full-time members include a trained general practitioner, a trained pediatric nurse, a pediatrician, a psychologist, and a social worker, and activities include identifying the needs of the child and the family in all dimensions in a standard way; managing symptoms in physical, mental, social, and spiritual dimensions; referral to other specialties as needed; counseling and follow-up; referral to other centers (home, general clinics, general hospital, or children's specialized hospital) as needed; child and family empowerment; training service providers in other covered centers; recording and documenting; conducting research and evaluating the services provided; and providing planning and policy making for the development of services.

In the form of independent centers (spokes), the general doctor and experienced nurse are the main and full-time members of the center, and activities include identifying the needs of the child and family, managing symptoms, referring to other centers as needed, 24-hour support for the child and family, and empowerment. The child and the family do registration and documentation and cooperate in conducting research by helping to collect information [22].

## 1.7 Pediatric Oncology Palliative Care Interdisciplinary Team and the Role of the Nurse

Palliative care is a service that is interdisciplinary in nature [23]. In an interdisciplinary team, various members work together, including doctors, nurses, social workers, psychologists, psychiatrists, nutritionists, rehabilitation specialists, and spiritual caregivers [24, 25]. In an interdisciplinary palliative care team, nurses play a key role [26] because they are often the first care providers and have the most contact with patients and families [27]. In order for a nurse to be able to provide services in an interdisciplinary pediatric oncology palliative care team, it is necessary to be qualified. In this regard, nurses who have a bachelor's degree, master's degree, or doctorate in nursing education, have at least 1 year of work experience in the pediatric oncology department, and are trained in the field of palliative care can work under titles such as "general nurse," "experienced nurse in the field of pediatric oncology," or "expert nurse in the field of pediatric palliative care" to provide services in an interdisciplinary team of pediatric oncology palliative care.

The duties of nurses in a pediatric oncology palliative care team and at different levels in Iran are as follows: basic level: villages and cities with a population of less than 20,000, level 1: cities with more than 20,000 people, level 2: cities with more than 50,000 people, level 3: cities Bogor and centers of the province. It is possible to fully examine the child and family based on standard tools, manage physical and mental symptoms at a mild to moderate level, plan to support the bereaved family, plan to support the child's sister/brother, plan for social support with Aid from charities and volunteers, spiritual support with the cooperation of spiritual care providers, family education and their empowerment, holding general training classes on palliative care in cancer in the covered population, empowering volunteers in child and family support, referral to other levels in case need, requesting various consultations such as psychology or nutrition [22].

## 1.8 Evaluating the Gap in Children's Palliative Care Provision

Evaluating the gap in children's palliative care is crucial for policy makers to comprehend the need and justify resource allocation. By identifying current children's palliative care services, it can also aid in developing better models of care within countries by recognizing successful practices, areas for improvement, and lessons learned. When mapping services, it is crucial to consider community- and hospital-based services, particularly in light of integration efforts such as the WHA resolution on palliative care, Universal Health Coverage (UHC), and the Astana Declaration. Several nations do not regularly gather specific indicators to evaluate service provision, and when indicators are collected, they often rely on proxies such as per capita morphine use. The development of indicators for mapping children's palliative care is expected to aid future in-country development [28].

## 1.9 Palliative Care in North of Iran

Regarding to improving the quality of life in cancer patients, WHO has announced in its recent statement on climate and cancer control that palliative care programs should be included in the university curriculum of the Mediterranean region, including Iran, and relevant training courses should be provided. The care provider should be held periodically and palliative care should be part of the national cancer control program in each country; in addition, the existence of regional and national guidelines for the implementation of palliative care is very necessary. In this regard, in Iran, numerous activities have been carried out, including training courses for interdisciplinary teams, the development of guidelines, research and publication and books, master's and doctoral theses, and the provision of palliative care for children and adults in several cases. A pilot hospital nationwide and the preparation of the initial statute for the formation of a palliative care association are among the activities carried out. Given the gaps in palliative care provision in Iran, a research project in the form of a doctoral thesis by one of the authors (S.P.) and supervised by the professors of this book (N.J.P. and Z.TE.) and other prominent professors, was conducted through participatory action research for two years from 2021 to 2023. The result of this research was the selection of the pediatric oncology department of the 17-Shahrivar Educational and Medical Center in Rasht (northern Iran) as the second center for providing palliative care in Iran after the Mofid Center in Tehran.

# 2 Communication

## 2.1 Communication and Communication Therapy

Communication is an exchange of facts, ideas, opinions, or emotions by two or more persons (Fig. 2.1).

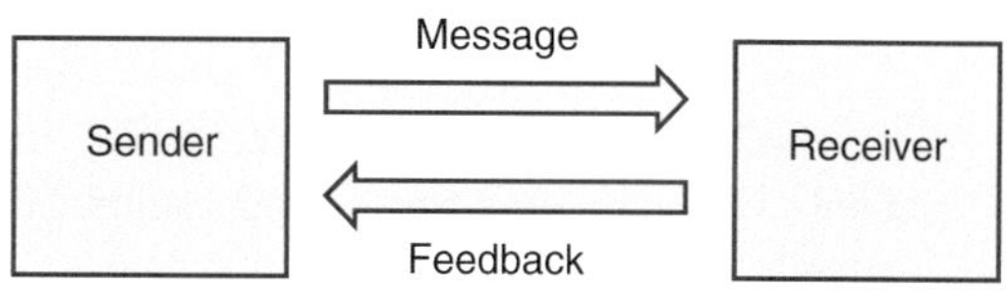


**Fig. 2.1** Communication process. This figure is researcher-made design and has not been adapted from any resource

Effective communication requires trust and mutual respect, which is very important in nursing, because communication is the basis of nursing activity [29]. Oncology nurses need to communicate with patients in the best way to obtain history and check and refer patients and families. This type of communication established between patient and nurse is called therapeutic communication. In this regard, familiarizing nurses with communication barriers is very beneficial.

Effective communication is crucial for providing quality palliative care, but it's important to recognize and address any difficulties that may arise. It always involves both parties, necessitating sensitivity, empathy, and active listening. Open communication can be hindered by societal attitudes toward death and dying. Health professionals may feel uneasy about death and dying, want to protect themselves and others, and experience discomfort with intense emotions. Busy health professionals often resort to blocking tactics that hinder communication, like prioritizing tasks over interaction [30]. Lack of privacy and adequate time and space to listen could create an additional hazard. The key to effective communication is our listening skills, not the words we use. Effective communication is crucial in palliative care to accurately assess patients' physical, emotional, and psychosocial needs. In order to support patients and families dealing with change and uncertainty, healthcare professionals must learn about patients' expectations and goals [23].

## 2.2 Challenges in Communication

Communication is hindered by different barriers [31].

### 2.2.1 Healthcare Professional-Led Barriers

Communication behavior can be influenced by four factors: fears, beliefs, inadequate skills, and lack of support.



N. Javadi-Pashaki et al., *Interdisciplinary Pediatric Palliative Care*,
https://doi.org/10.1007/978-981-97-9587-1_2

### Fears

- About releasing intense feelings.
- The risk of upsetting the patient outweighs the potential benefits.
- Dealing with unanswerable and challenging questions, like "why me?"
- Risking trouble with the HCP hierarchy by saying the wrong thing.
- Spending an excessive amount of time.
- Handling emotional reactions from patients.

### Beliefs

- Emotional problems are unavoidable in patients with serious diseases and cannot be resolved.
- Certain matters are not within my jurisdiction to discuss. Senior team members need to be involved in these discussions.
- Discussing fears is pointless without any answers.
- Discussing unsolvable concerns only leads to false hope.

### Inadequate Skills

- Unsure how to evaluate knowledge and perceptions
- The inability to incorporate medical, psychological, social, and spiritual aspects
- Lacking knowledge on navigating emotions securely
- Uncertain about how to navigate challenging communication scenarios like delivering bad news or managing anger

### Lack of Support

- If problems were identified, the patient felt unsupported.
- The HCP may feel unsupported.
- There is a conflict among team members [31].

## 2.2.2 Patient-Led Barriers

Only 40% of patients disclose their concerns, and the most anxious or distressed reveal the least. Patient non-disclosure reasons mirror professional-led obstacles like fears, beliefs, and other challenges.

### Fears

- Acknowledging the inability to handle a situation.
- Losing composure in front of unfamiliar people.
- Admitting psychological problems can lead to stigmatization.
- The confirmation of their worst fears.
- Striving to safeguard staff from their suffering.

### Beliefs

- Healthcare professionals are seen as excessively occupied.
- The HCP's focus is limited to specific areas of care, like nurses with physical care and doctors with disease and treatment concerns.
- The burden for healthcare professionals will be greater with the increase in talking concerns.
- Life relies on receiving treatment, and complaining about it will result in its removal. "I mustn't alienate or upset the doctor."

### Difficulties

- They are unable to put their feelings into words. The consultation might have overwhelmed them, causing them to forget their main concern.
- I can't seem to find the correct words. They might not be familiar with the technical language as well as the concepts of disease evolution and spread.

- Healthcare professionals have been responding to their concerns with distancing when they try to express them.
- Lacks sufficient language skills and lacks access to an independent interpreter.
- The professional fails to ask the appropriate questions [31].

**There are some other barriers as below:**

Giving advice: Sometimes giving advice gives the opposite result. The patient/caregiver says I'm bored. Nurse's answer: Go outside for a walk (wrong); what is the cause of your impatience? Explain to me, maybe I can help you (correct).

Judging: Outright judgment leads to loss of trust of the patient/companion. Saying phrases like "You are wrong" or "What you are doing for your sick child is not right" is wrong, and you should say "Well, your interpretation is different, I want to know your point of view on this matter and talk to me."

Reassuring: Giving the patient/family false hope is deceiving and is a major communication barrier. For example, a child has cancer and the parents ask the nurse, "Will my child get well?" And the nurse says "it will be fine, don't worry" (wrong). The correct answer is: "We will do everything we can for your child and trust in God."

Repetitive or stereotyped answers: For example, regarding everything the patient/family says, use a sentence like "Your doctor knows what medicine to prescribe" instead of listening to the patient/family, which gives the patient this feeling. He conveys that the nurse does not want to listen to his words. Or, in some cases, the patient should not be asked a question that the answer of "no" or "yes" by the patient will cause disruption in the treatment. For example, if you ask the patient: "Are you ready to get out of bed and the patient answers yes, in the event that he must get off the bed and otherwise it will cause problems for him, you have actually given him the opportunity to say no." But in some cases, it is necessary to use only questions that have a yes or no answer, for example, "Do you feel pain when I move your arm like this?" It also causes the fear of the patient, for example, "How come you haven't made a decision to pursue your child's treatment yet?" Here, it is better to ask, "What makes your decision to pursue your child's treatment stronger?"

Hostility or taking a defensive posture: At all times, the nurse should be tolerant and avoid getting angry in front of any patient or companions. For example, instead of using words such as "You shouldn't have spoken like this," use words such as "This experience must be very difficult for you," so that the patient feels comfortable and expresses his anxiety easily.

Imposing values: The nurse should not impose his personal values and opinions on the patient. For example, avoid using sentences like "You were wrong to do that" or "If I were in your place." Also, guiding questions should be avoided, for example, the nurse says: You don't want to smoke this cigarette anymore, don't you? Instead of making the patient say whatever is on his mind, this prayer directly induces the feeling to the patient that the patient is expected to say what the nurse expects.

Rejecting: Rejecting, consciously or unconsciously, causes disconnection. Saying things like "You shouldn't feel this way" or "I don't want to hear these things" conveys the idea that the patient is worthless. This method is effective even in non-verbal communication. For example, turning one's face away from a patient and looking behind one's eyes are examples of rejection.

Judging expressions: The cause of the abuse of nursing standards toward the patient, pay attention to this phrase that was said by the nurse to a crying mother: "Your action shows your immaturity. How can you not think?" How will your husband feel when he sees you crying like this? In this situation, the nurse judges that the mother has a child with minor cancer and the obvious opposition can cause the effective communication to be cut off. Instead, it is better to say "I would like to help you. Tell me what made you cry?" Or the patient says: "I think I'm right that I don't feel afraid of this surgery" and the nurse says "Tell me what made you afraid?" In this case, the patient is allowed to talk about his feelings without any judgment. Here, the nurse must show her agreement or disagreement with the help of others.

### 2.2.3 How to Deal with Aggressive Patients/Companions?

At first, one should avoid approaching the patient or his companions, because this behavior leads to more aggression and irritation.

After knowing the factors that provoke the anger of the patient/companions, efforts should be made to understand him and give him the opportunity to express his problem by talking. In this regard, sympathy with the patient is helpful. For example, say: "You look angry." "What's your problem?/Why are you angry? Let's talk about your problem." These conversations allow the patient or companions to talk about their problem and vent.

Talk to the patient/family in a way that shows that you welcome them warmly.

Tell angry patient/companions "We will do whatever we can for you and we are by your side" or "We will do whatever we can to help you."

Since the angry patient/partner does not think very logically, it is better that you do not talk too much or that your sentences are not complicated.

Staff who have little patience should not talk to an angry patient/companion, because their anger leads to more anger in the patient/companion.

Don't gossip or chat with your colleagues.

What to do in critical situations when dealing with aggressive patients/companions?

- Be as calm as you can and tell the patient/patient's companion to be calm and let's talk about your problem together.
- Do not humiliate or make fun of the patient/companions.
- Encourage patient/companions to sit and talk.
- Ask them to talk about their situation (anger, etc.).
- Cut off the surrounding sounds (television, etc.) and speak slowly and don't get angry. Do not shout loudly.
- Do not make eye contact with angry patient/companions as much as possible in critical situations.
- Avoid expressions such as "why are you yelling," "why are you acting like a child," or "what are you doing?" [32].

## 2.3 Communication Skills

Key communication skills are:

**Active Listening: Paying Attention to What the Other Person Is Saying**

- Not interrupting conversations and making hasty decisions
- Reflecting the person's speech and providing feedback
- Repeating the feedback process to ensure correct understanding of the other person's words

**Sympathy**

- Ability to understand the situation of the other person
- Correctly understanding the feelings of the other person
- Showing the other person that we put ourselves in his place

**Empathy**

Describing the other person's feelings or situation and specifying expectations from each other [33]

### 2.3.1 Important Points in Communicating with the Child

- In communicating with children, we should use appropriate solutions according to their age.
- Things like giving independence to the child, providing self-esteem, and creating psychological security in children are very effective in establishing effective communication.
- Explaining to the child/adolescent about the diagnostic and therapeutic procedures (examination, injection, etc.) in simple and understandable language and appropriate to the level of development and cognitive understanding of the child/adolescent before performing the work/procedure.
- Not threatening or scaring the child
- Not saying phrases like "If you don't cooperate with us or don't let me examine you, your illness will get worse" or "If you don't let me inject you with this medicine, your condition will get worse" or "If you don't let me give you your medicine, I won't let your parents give you today."
- Reassuring the child about the presence of parents by their side and their supporting role.
- Explanation about your support ("I'm by your side and you don't have to worry at all").
- Educating parents before invasive diagnostic or therapeutic procedures.
- No separation of the child/adolescent from the parents except in special circumstances.
- Telling the truth to parents along with honesty and empathy and supporting them.
- Obtaining permission from the parents and the child/adolescent before performing any diagnostic and therapeutic measures (especially physical examinations related to genital organs, etc.).
- If the child is immature, get help from female staff for handling, injections, etc. and, if the child is older or a teenager, from staff of the same sex.
- In the department, there should be toys, books, and magazines suitable for the child's age. Play equipment should be clean, standard, and suitable for the child's developmental age and can be used to show hospital activities (such as injections, examination, taking medicine, etc.). You can use things like toys as a reward for the good behavior of children.
- Important points in respecting the rights of children and families.
- Care regardless of age, gender, race, or ethnicity and cultural beliefs.
- Obtaining informed consent and voluntary participation in research projects.
- Taking photos or videos after obtaining written consent.
- Confidentiality of the child's medical information.
- Treating the child and family politely.
- Presenting the prognosis of the disease and the treatments available in this center with empathy and simple expression (first we explain to the parents in simple and understandable language and then the parents explain to their child. Finally, the nurse explains to the child in simple language).
- Having the right to make decisions about diagnostic-therapeutic methods after providing complete information by the nurse and physician.
- Performing the procedures if it is associated with the least pain of the child/adolescent.
- Children who are hospitalized in adult hospitals should be in a separate room and ward, and all equipment such as the possibility of education, games, etc. should be provided for them.
- Anger, blaming yourself and the medical staff, and depression are common problems in parents with hospitalized children [34, 35].

## 2.4 Breaking Bad News

Bad news refers to any information about the patient's illness that is perceived negatively by society and the patient. Making informed choices and future plans requires attentive listening and thoughtful responses. Attending to cultural and language barriers and addressing strong emotions are crucial for holistic palliative care.

In cases where the patient cannot make decisions about their illness, such as when experiencing consciousness disorder or acute psychotic attack, as well as mentally disabled patients and underage children, a legal substitute is appointed to handle their affairs [36].

### 2.4.1 The Goals of Breaking Bad News

Breaking bad news must be customized to address the unique needs of each person, considering their individual history and fears. Breaking bad news should be done in a manner that promotes acceptance and understanding while minimizing negative reactions. Mastering the art of delivering bad news requires honed and updated skills, comparable to a surgeon's dedication to their craft. If the process is performed poorly, it can have immediate and long-lasting negative consequences for everyone involved, just like a failed surgery. For example, patients and families may lose trust. Knowing how to effectively complete the process is important, but delivering bad news should never feel routine or lacking in compassion [37–39].

### 2.4.2 Approaches of Breaking Bad News

- SPIKES
- ABCDE
- BREAKS [40]

### 2.4.3 What Is the SPIKES Approach?

- Place of presentation of bad news (setting): It should be in a quiet room and away from noise or traffic. Privacy should be respected. There are enough seats to sit. Reception facilities as well as necessary facilities to manage possible physiological reactions such as fainting of the patient, etc. should be available in the environment.
- Checking the patient's perception of his condition (perception of condition): Check the patient's knowledge about his disease. Does the patient/family know the status/severity of their cancer? Listen to the patient/family. Accept patient/family denial at this point.
- Giving information to the patient/family (invitation to give information): Ask the patient/family if they would like to have more information about their condition. The reluctance of the patient/family to receive more information should be respected.
- Telling the facts to the patient (knowledge: giving medical facts): In this step, the facts of the disease should be told to the person in simple language and taking into account the literacy level, socio-cultural situation, and current emotional state. At first, you should mention the positive aspects of the disease (e.g., fortunately, the cancer has not spread to the lymph nodes, this type of cancer is highly treatable, and treatments for this type of cancer are easily accessible at this center). Give the information to the patient in a short and concise manner and check whether he understood what you said or not. In the following, all the facts related to the disease, the type of treatments available, and the prognosis should be presented to the patient. Also try to give a suitable answer to the reactions of the patients.
- Empathy with the patient (explore emotions and sympathize): In this step, you should identify the patient's emotions and their cause (sadness, discomfort, shock) and then give the patient time to express his emotions. Finally, you must respond to these emotions in such a way that the patient realizes that you understand him completely.
- Summary and conclusion of the session (strategy and summary): In this step, the session will end and ask the patient if there are any questions left for him or not. Also, talk to him about the next meeting (e.g., I will talk to you again when the results of the follow-up tests are ready) [37].

Note: The doctor in charge of the patient, who is the most knowledgeable person in the treatment team, is responsible for telling the bad news to the patient or his companion [37].

### 2.4.4 How Do People React to Receiving Bad News?

- Shock
- Denial
- Anger
- Disappointment to the future
- Blaming yourself and family
- Restlessness
- Feeling guilty and guilty

### 2.4.5 What Are the Precautions After Announcing the Bad News to People?

- All reactions of patients and families (such as anger, denial, hopelessness, guilt, or despair) after receiving bad news are normal and should not be ignored.
- Guide the patient and family to a quiet room and allow them to sit down and maintain their privacy.
- Allow the patient and family to talk, cry, and express their anger.
- Do not stop their crying or anger.
- Give the patient and family time to face the reality.
- Let the patient and family talk.
- Be a good listener for them.
- Pay attention to the non-verbal gestures of the patient and the family [41].

### 2.4.6 Handling Difficult Questions

For example, "Is it cancer? Am I dying? What is going to happen to me?"

**Key Points**

- Determine the patient's beliefs regarding the reasons behind their question: "What makes you think it might be cancer or that you're dying?"
- If needed, ask if there are any other reasons for the patient feeling this way, after receiving a response.
- **If the patient gives no other reason or changes the subject:**

  You might say: "Would you like to discuss the diagnosis you asked about?" If the patient declines, respect their decision and move on [41].
- **If the patient gives other reasons:**

  Validate the patient's thoughts if they are accurate. If appropriate, offer support and encourage the patient to share their emotions. Take a moment to see if the patient brings up any concerns on their own. If that's not the case, encourage the patient to express their worries. It is wise to focus on the concerns raised by the patient. Nevertheless, respond truthfully and avoid hastily providing premature or false reassurances.
- Feel free to ask any additional questions.
- I can provide you with relevant information, either written or verbal.
- When conceptualization is challenging, drawings can be useful. Patients only need a clearly written disease or complication name to remember. They will probably seek advice from friends and use the Internet to ensure consistent care. This will also involve extending access for discussion, similar to when delivering unfortunate news. A near future contingency plan may be part of it as well [41].

### 2.4.7 Collusion

This can happen when a healthcare professional is pressured by a relative to hide medical information from the patient. The HCP is being asked to conspire with the relative to hide or lie about the seriousness of the patient's illness. The reason often given is that the relative has a deep understanding of the patient and believes they would simply give up. In another scenario, they would struggle to handle the truth and the relative sees no reason for the patient to worry about bad news.

Concentrate on these key points:

- The emotions of the family member.
- The reasons why the relative doesn't want to be honest.
- Acknowledging the relative's motives, e.g., protecting the patient from distress.

- Taking into account the relative's intentions, like safeguarding the patient from distress.
- How the relative perceives the patient's understanding. Look for any signs that the patient may already suspect the truth.

Then:

- Offer to directly evaluate the patient's comprehension of their condition.
- Assure the family member that the patient won't receive any information unless they explicitly ask for it [42].

### 2.4.8 Dealing with Anger

**Key Points**

- These strategies are effective in calming anger:
  Recognize the anger by saying "You appear to be extremely angry," which might temporarily intensify their anger. This is particularly true when their anger is directed toward you. If there's no opportunity to express it, anger won't go away.
- I would appreciate it if you could help me understand the reason behind your anger.
- Gather as much information as possible by listening to their story.
- Don't get defensive, even if the anger seems to be aimed at the wrong target. The person who expresses anger often realizes the unfairness of displacement.
- Pay attention to the person's stress and emotions.
- If necessary, apologize, but there's no need to apologize for something that clearly isn't your fault or responsibility.
- If it's appropriate, clarify the situation by acknowledging how difficult it must be for you to see your husband in pain.
- If it is feasible, engage in negotiations to reach a solution that is acceptable to both parties. This might involve acknowledging the unacceptability of a specific situation and guiding the individual toward the appropriate channels for filing a complaint [41, 43, 44].

# 3 Grief

## 3.1 Grief Definition

Grief is a cognitive, emotional, psychological, and physical reaction that follows the loss of anything dear and important to us. It is a natural reaction to the loss of something dear to us [45].

Bereavement that is officially recognized somewhere, such as grief due to the separation of a spouse, grief due to the death of a classmate or friend, and grief.

Grief experienced by a community following a common event such as pandemics and war.

Anticipatory grief and bereavement encompass various dimensions including physical, psychological, spiritual, social, and cultural aspects. According to the definition provided by Webster's Dictionary, "bereaved" is a term derived from the words "reaved" or "reft," which signify the act of depriving and causing desolation, particularly through death. The experience of bereavement is a lifelong journey characterized by fluctuations. The central element is the child, encircled by concentric spheres of family, friends, professionals, and the broader community and culture [23].

Both the experience of anticipatory grief and bereavement in children necessitate the presence of honesty, reassurance, and a secure outlet for emotional expression. The occurrence of death disrupts a child's perception that the world is secure and predictable, where misfortunes are limited to those who deserve them, where virtuous behavior is rewarded, and where a higher power can provide solace and improvement [46]. Following the revelation of a potentially life-threatening illness in a child by a medical professional, one of the most challenging tasks a parent will face is to carry on this conversation with the affected child and other siblings within the family. The disclosure and ensuing conversation evoke anticipatory grief, a significant and inherent process that arises throughout the child's lifetime. This process serves to prepare both the child and the family for the inevitability of dying and death. Following the passing, the grieving individuals undergo the journey of bereavement and experience the healing process of grief. Bereavement is a transformative journey through which the grieving individuals strive to incorporate the departed into their future endeavors, rather than simply leaving them behind. This serves as a means to ensure that the memory of the deceased remains alive and that forthcoming generations will have a sense of familiarity with them.

The provision of honesty, reassurance, and a safe space for emotional expression is necessary when offering support for children experiencing anticipatory grief and bereavement. The disclosure of a diagnosis of a life-threatening condition (LTC) initiates anticipatory grief, which serves to prepare the child and family for the process of dying and death. The process of bereavement encompasses a broad spectrum of emotions, experiences, thoughts, physical symptoms, social



N. Javadi-Pashaki et al., *Interdisciplinary Pediatric Palliative Care*,
https://doi.org/10.1007/978-981-97-9587-1_3

adjustments, and spiritual changes that occur over an extended duration, occurring at different intervals and with varying degrees of intensity and combinations.

Children and young individuals who have experienced loss require empathetic listening, as well as permission and guidance to mourn in their own distinct manner. They should be assured that there is no correct or incorrect way to grieve and provided with adequate time and support to express their emotions [30]. The fundamental principles of anticipatory grief and bereavement encompass:

- The experience of anticipatory grief and bereavement, which encompass the periods before and after the loss, commences upon the child's diagnosis and continues for years following their passing.
- Anticipatory grief is the expression of sorrow when a loss is perceived as inevitable or threatening.
- A child mourns for every person and thing in their life.
- The family experiences collective losses prior to the child's passing, followed by the grieving process.
- The child and family might experience a sense of being overwhelmed by the intensity of their emotions, without realizing that underlying their feelings of sadness is the more profound concept of anticipatory grief. Clarifying this distinction can be of relief and comfort.
- The passing of another patient brings about profound sorrow and anticipatory grief for both the sick children and their families who are grieving.
- A lifelong process characterized by fluctuations. There is no definitive timeline for the resolution of this matter.
- Families frequently experience a dual sense of loss: both for their child as an individual and as a member of their family and community and for their professional family—the team that provided care for the child, often for extended periods of time.
- The inclusion of bereavement follow-up is essential in providing comprehensive pediatric palliative care and addresses the family's feelings of abandonment.
- The assessment and subsequent reassessment of bereavement serve as both a preventive measure and an intervention.
- Despite experiencing the loss of the same child, family members undergo the grieving process in distinct manners and at varying intervals. Experiencing a lack of synchronization is a common occurrence.
- Siblings experience profound grief over the loss of their brother or sister. Nevertheless, due to the significant differences in the ways children express grief compared to adults, their mourning may be undervalued or overlooked entirely [47].

- Pain and guilt
- Anger and bargaining
- Depression and loneliness
- Acceptance and hope [48]

Grieving involves three key concepts: loss, grief, and mourning. Loss refers to the absence of something valuable or anticipated, eliciting grief and expressed through mourning. It can pertain to losing health, altered relationships, shifting roles, or life itself. After someone passes away, their loved ones face the profound impact of loss [49]. Grief, however, is an emotional reaction to loss, deeply personal and unique to each individual. It encompasses feelings like sadness, anger, guilt, loneliness, and even peace, affecting people physically, emotionally, socially, and spiritually. Grief does not follow a linear process; it is unpredictable, with moments of acceptance alternating with periods of deep pain. Mourning is the outward expression of loss, shaped by cultural norms, rituals, and traditions. It varies widely—some cultures encourage vocal expressions like crying, while others lean toward stoic responses. Personality and life experiences also influence how mourning is displayed [50].

## 3.2 Types of Grief

There are five types of grief: anticipatory grief, acute grief, normal grief, disenfranchised grief, and complicated grief:

### 3.2.1 Anticipatory Grief

Anticipatory grief occurs before a loss, often linked to a terminal diagnosis or major life changes. Patients may grieve over lost independence or missed future milestones, while families grieve the impending absence of their loved ones. This form of grief can help ease the emotional shock of bereavement [51].

### 3.2.2 Acute Grief

Acute grief begins immediately after a loss, marked by disbelief, confusion, and a temporary disengagement from daily life as the reality of separation sets in [50].

### 3.2.3 Normal Grief

Normal grief includes typical emotional, physical, cognitive, and behavioral responses to loss. While intense, it gradually eases, allowing individuals to reconnect with life, even though the loss remains a part of them [50].

### 3.2.4 Disenfranchised Grief

Disenfranchised grief arises when a loss is not socially acknowledged or validated. This may occur with stigmatized losses, such as deaths related to illness or terminated pregnancies, leaving individuals unable to mourn openly.

### 3.2.5 Complicated Grief

Complicated grief affects a minority of people, with intense, prolonged reactions to loss. It includes subtypes like chronic grief (persistent and unresolved), delayed grief (postponed emotional reactions), exaggerated grief (extreme reactions like phobias or suicidal thoughts), and masked grief (unrecognized behaviors stemming from grief). Risk factors include traumatic deaths, unresolved past losses, and inadequate support systems, often necessitating professional intervention. Each type of grief reflects the complex ways humans respond to loss, emphasizing the need for compassionate support tailored to individual experiences [50].

## 3.3 Stages of Grief

Grief often unfolds in stages following a loss. Nurses benefit from understanding these stages, as it helps them recognize emotional reactions as natural parts of grief and provide better support to patients and families coping with loss. Renowned Swiss psychiatrist Elisabeth Kübler-Ross outlined five primary stages of grief in her book *On Death and Dying* [52]. These stages—denial, anger, bargaining, depression, and acceptance—are remembered by the acronym "DABDA." Grieving individuals may experience these stages in a fluid and non-linear manner, moving back and forth between them, skipping some stages, or experiencing them in a different order. Since there is no single "right" way to grieve, care plans must be tailored to the unique needs and emotions of each person. The Kübler-Ross model highlights that grief responses are not limited to the loss of life; they can also result from major life changes, such as divorce, job loss, the end of a friendship, or receiving a diagnosis of a chronic or terminal illness [53]. (Refer to Fig. 3.1 for a visual representation of the Kübler-Ross grief cycle.)

### 3.3.1 Denial

Denial occurs when individuals refuse to acknowledge a loss or act as though it is not happening. This self-protective mechanism helps them cope with the shock of overwhelm-

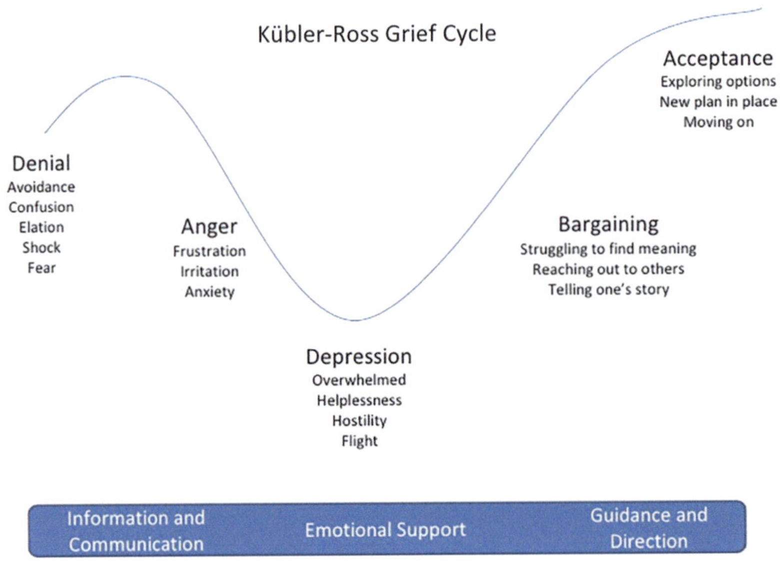


**Fig. 3.1** Kübler-Ross grief cycle. (Source: Reprinted with permission from "Kubler-ross-grief-cycle-1-728.jpg" by U3173699 is licensed under CC BY-SA 4.0)

ing emotions by temporarily numbing the pain. Commonly expressed as "This can't be happening," denial often arises during traumatic or unexpected losses or following unforeseen life-changing events. For instance, a patient diagnosed with terminal brain cancer after seeking help for severe headaches might experience denial as a way to process the devastating news.

### 3.3.2 Anger

Anger often emerges during grief as a way to mask underlying pain and sadness. This anger may be directed toward the deceased, oneself, or others and can sometimes seem misdirected or without clear cause. In health care settings, anger may be aimed at caregivers or medical professionals as a reaction to the situation, not as a personal attack. Recognizing this can help caregivers provide support while maintaining boundaries for respectful communication. Nurses can create a safe space for patients or families to express their emotions, allowing them to vent frustration and sorrow without judgment.

### 3.3.3 Bargaining

Bargaining is an attempt to regain a sense of control over the loss by negotiating or making promises to change the circumstances. This stage often involves pleas to a higher power, such as a patient saying, "I'll stop smoking if God heals my wife's cancer." Through bargaining, individuals seek a way to alter their reality, even if the loss is inevitable.

### 3.3.4 Depression

Depression in grief manifests as intense sadness over the loss, often leading to withdrawal from activities, people, and relationships. Common symptoms include irritability, sleeplessness, fatigue, and an overwhelming sense of despair. Everyday tasks, like getting out of bed or preparing a meal, can feel insurmountable. During this phase, individuals may struggle to find meaning or self-worth. Nurses should monitor for ineffective coping behaviors, such as self-medication with alcohol or drugs, and provide appropriate support or resources.

### 3.3.5 Acceptance

Acceptance involves understanding and acknowledging the loss while recognizing the ability to cope with it. This phase does not eliminate sadness but reflects an adjustment to the new reality. Individuals begin to reconnect with others, establish new routines, and rediscover moments of happiness and purpose [53].

## 3.4 Grief Tasks

In addition to the stages of grief outlined by Kübler-Ross, other experts describe the grieving process in terms of tasks that individuals must navigate.

### 3.4.1 Notification and Shock

This initial phase involves acknowledging the reality of the loss. Individuals may feel numb or isolated while processing the news.

### 3.4.2 Experiencing the Loss

The second task focuses on emotional and cognitive engagement with the loss. This involves expressing and working through the pain of separation and grief.

### 3.4.3 Reintegration

In this final task, individuals reorganize their lives and relationships, adapting to an environment without the deceased. This includes forming a new reality while cherishing memories of the lost loved one. As a nurse, you can support grieving patients and families by offering your presence, listening to their stories, and validating their emotions. While you cannot resolve their grief, assessing their needs and providing resources can help guide them through the process [51].

## 3.5 Bereavement

Bereavement encompasses the inner feelings of grief and the outward expressions of mourning experienced after the death of a loved one. The bereavement period refers to the time it takes for an individual to process the pain of loss, grieve, mourn, and adapt to life without the deceased. This process can have significant physical impacts, including an elevated risk of myocardial infarction and cardiomyopathy. Widows and widowers, in particular, face a higher likelihood of death following the loss of a spouse. Encouraging bereaved individuals to talk openly about their loss and normalize their emotions is vital. They should allow themselves time to grieve and avoid making major decisions, such as relocating or changing jobs, during this period. Focusing on spirituality can also help them cope effectively. American culture often tends to suppress the expression of grief and the pain associated with loss, but experiencing and expressing these emotions is critical for healing. Nurses play a key role in supporting individuals during bereavement by:

- Enhancing coping strategies
- Supporting spiritual exploration
- Facilitating the grieving process by encouraging individuals to feel and express their loss while navigating the tasks of grief
- Communicating with the interdisciplinary care team to provide comprehensive support [50]

## 3.6 Children and Grief

Children experience grief uniquely, depending on their developmental stage, and may display either normal or complicated grief. Their ability to articulate their emotions is often limited, which can lead to behavioral and emotional manifestations.

- Younger children may exhibit symptoms such as nervousness, frequent illnesses, hyperactivity, nightmares, anger, dependency on a surviving parent, or denial. They may not grasp the permanence of death until around preschool age or older, making it essential to use clear language like "death" instead of euphemisms.

- Older children might experience difficulties such as trouble concentrating, declining academic performance, insomnia, social withdrawal, depression, rebellious behavior, suicidal thoughts, or experimenting with drugs or alcohol. Using therapeutic play can help children express their grief in a way they understand. Nurses should reassure children that their feelings are normal and refer them and their families to grief specialists or local support groups as needed [50].

## 3.7 Parents and Grandparents

The death of a child is an overwhelming loss for parents, requiring substantial bereavement support. For grandparents, the grief is often compounded by witnessing their child's (the parent's) sorrow, and their own grief is frequently overlooked [50].

## 3.8 Completion of the Grieving Process

Grief is not a process that has a definitive endpoint, as certain triggers—such as memories, objects, songs, or anniversaries—can rekindle feelings of loss. However, healing occurs when:

- The pain of the loss diminishes.
- The individual adapts to life without the deceased.
- The person achieves physical, psychological, and social "letting go." Letting go is a challenging yet necessary process. It involves accepting the loss while still cherishing the love and meaning of the relationship. Importantly, letting go does not mean severing ties with memories but rather finding ways to adapt and maintain meaningful connections with the deceased [50].

## 3.9 Self-Care for Nurses

End-of-life care can profoundly affect nurses, especially when patient loss is sudden, traumatic, or occurs repeatedly. For example, an emergency room nurse handling the death of a child from an accident may find it difficult to cope with such a loss. Repeated exposure to loss, particularly in high-stress situations such as during the COVID-19 pandemic, can result in compassion fatigue and burnout.

- Compassion fatigue refers to chronic self-sacrifice and prolonged exposure to emotionally taxing situations, which can harm physical, emotional, and spiritual well-being.
- Burnout manifests as physical and emotional exhaustion, reduced motivation, and a sense of cynicism. It is often triggered by overwhelming workplace demands, resource shortages, or interpersonal and policy-related stressors [50].

## 3.10 Preventing Compassion Fatigue and Burnout

Self-care is essential to address and prevent these challenges. Nurses are encouraged to:

- Take time off when needed.
- Develop healthy coping mechanisms such as prayer, meditation, exercise, art, or music.
- Utilize organizational support, such as employee assistance programs offering counseling or debriefing sessions led by chaplains. By participating in these sessions, nurses can openly express their feelings and process losses in a supportive environment [50].

## 3.11 Self-Assessment and Awareness

To recognize early signs of compassion fatigue and burnout, nurses should reflect on questions such as:

- Have my behaviors or communication patterns changed?
- Am I engaging in destructive habits?
- Do I project my internal struggles onto others?

Self-awareness allows nurses to implement strategies to manage stress [50]. Building resilience with the four "A's."

- Attention: Monitor your physical, emotional, social, and spiritual well-being. Reflect on what you are grateful for and areas where you can improve.
- Acknowledgment: Confront and accept the losses you have witnessed, finding meaning in the experiences.
- Affection: Show kindness and warmth toward yourself, avoiding self-criticism or bitterness.
- Acceptance: Embrace all aspects of yourself, including your talents and imperfections, fostering peace and patience. By prioritizing self-care and seeking professional development, such as obtaining a palliative care certification, nurses can enhance their resilience and effectiveness in providing compassionate care while maintaining their well-being [50].

## 3.12 The Process of Bereavement

### 3.12.1 Fundamentals of Bereavement Assessment

#### 3.12.1.1 Assessment

In optimal conditions, a mental health clinician conducts a thorough assessment of bereavement. However, other scenarios are possible. In cases where a family feels more at ease with a different team member, that individual can serve as a facilitator by introducing and emphasizing the significance of the assessment. The effective execution of bereavement assessments can be achieved through the collaboration of an interdisciplinary pair, consisting of a medical professional and a psychological expert. In instances where a mental health clinician is unavailable for direct clinical engagement, an alternate team member may conduct the assessment and subsequently seek consultation regarding the family's status, risk, and needs. The evaluation for bereavement is typically conducted through multiple sessions, commencing in certain cases shortly after the child's passing and subsequently continuing for weeks or even months. The clinician must diligently observe the tempo of the assessment, both during meetings and in scheduling future appointments, always taking into account the family's cues. Rushing through an interview solely to meet the assessment requirements often leads to distress and the omission of crucial information. Following the child's death, it is crucial to evaluate the response of each family member and identify the necessary measures to support the family during this crisis. This may involve providing referrals for medical or mental health concerns. In the preliminary discussions, individuals frequently express their preferences regarding funeral and/or memorial services, as well as burial arrangements. In certain cases, logistical matters pertaining to body transportation may also be addressed. In cases where the family has not made prior arrangements, they frequently require support in navigating their available choices. The initial assessment may also involve a delicate examination of the family's financial assets and identification of individuals who can provide assistance during the upcoming days and weeks. Inquiries concerning the child's illness progression and demise, as well as any unresolved matters with the medical staff, are typically better addressed post the service. Additional significant aspects of bereavement assessment involve considering the individual's developmental stage and the family dynamics. The term "loss history" encompasses a wide range of losses. For instance, one may encounter these difficulties through illness, death, trauma, or alterations in relationships (like divorce). An essential aspect of the loss history encompasses the experiences of immigrant or refugee families. Alongside the loss of their home country, many have endured indescribable trauma during their journey to their new residence. Considering the highly sensitive nature of these issues, which may involve concerns about legal ramifications when disclosed, it is crucial to approach any inquiry with the utmost care. The core of the bereavement assessment revolves around the family's encounter with the child's illness and subsequent passing. Prior to addressing this portion of the interview, it is advisable to first invite the family to provide a description and engage in reminiscence of their child. It is crucial to hear the family's narrative as they choose to retell it, as it holds value in both its substance and manner of delivery. It is crucial to pay attention to and encourage the family to express both the facts and the associated emotions regarding the following matters:

- How was the communication of information about your child relayed to you?
- How did you and the staff communicate information to your child?
- Were you and your child involved in the decision-making process regarding treatment?
- Did you experience any particular ease or discomfort with any member of the staff?
- Could you please share the circumstances and timing surrounding your realization or notification of your child's impending demise?
- Were you provided with information regarding home and hospice options and comfort measures for your child?
- Were you adequately prepared for the anticipated circumstances surrounding the occurrence of death?
- Was the child exhibiting signs of distress prior to their passing?
- Prior to the death of your child, were there any instances where your family was the only ones present with them?
- Were you adequately supported by the staff?

Indicators of a potential challenging mourning period within a family may include a track record of multiple losses or traumatic events, psychiatric disturbances (particularly suicidal thoughts or behaviors), and substance dependencies. Family relationships that were previously delicate or strained are susceptible to further deterioration following the child's demise. In the event that the individual or family has an established connection with a mental health clinician, the team may request consent to communicate with said individual in order to facilitate prompt follow-up. It is crucial for individuals to ensure they have an emergency plan that encompasses immediate access to psychiatric assessment in the event of the child's death. The significance of assisting a family in establishing a network of extended family and friends as a "safety net" prior to the child's passing cannot be overstated. The assessment process operates on the foundational principle of always inquiring rather than assuming. Furthermore, the assessment serves as an initial stage in engaging with a grieving family, with the evaluation process persisting. Regularly checking in with one's family establishes consistent and supportive communication while also enabling the observation of potential emotional or behavioral changes that might otherwise go unnoticed. As an illustration, a parent might experience intermittent phases of appearing "almost normal," only to be accompanied by overwhelming sorrow, rendering them unable to leave their residence or even rise from bed. An additional instance could involve a sibling who seemingly functions normally but is suddenly afflicted by nightmares, becomes inconsolable and fearful, and withdraws from social interactions and hobbies. Examining the ethnic and cultural heritage, as well as the level of acculturation within immigrant families, is imperative for the evaluation and development of an ideal bereavement care strategy. There can be significant differences among family members in their adherence to beliefs and customs from their country of origin. Critical issues include:

- What are the familial beliefs and values regarding childhood illness and mortality?
- Is it deemed acceptable to discuss the topic of death in the presence of or with children?
- What are the patients' expectations regarding medical care and their level of engagement?
- What are the distinct and anticipated responsibilities of family members and the community?
- Are varying degrees of acculturation contributing to tension within familial relationships?

By conducting a comprehensive and meticulous investigation, valuable insights can be obtained to contextualize the psychological reactions of the family within their cultural heritage. The clinician's endeavor to comprehend these factors fosters a sense of respect and openness in the therapeutic alliance.

#### 3.12.1.2 Intervention

Currently, there is a lack of universally accepted standards for follow-up in pediatric palliative care related to bereavement. In the absence of individuals, it becomes imperative to prioritize the role of individual and family assessment, both in delivering optimal clinical care and in devising empirically testable protocols. The continuous assessment and reassessment process provides guidance to the clinician regarding the most valuable intervention at a given moment (Fig. 4.1). In order to achieve optimal "fit," a referral must be made based on careful clinical assessment, taking into account the specific needs and preferences of the individual or family. It is a common occurrence for these needs to change over time; therefore, a range of support and treatment methods may be utilized simultaneously or consecutively during the grieving process. Numerous families rely on their local community for assistance. As an illustration, a profoundly religious family may seek comfort through their spiritual institution. Some individuals seek support from self-help bereavement groups offered by local agencies, which depend on volunteers and trained peer counselors. Certain individuals opt for a more comprehensive approach by engaging in individual, marital, or family psychotherapy to explore the lasting effects of their child's illness and demise on their lives. Psychotherapy plays a crucial role in supporting individuals or families with pre-existing or current vulnerabilities that are connected to or inseparable from the loss of a child. The exact definition of "pathological grief" is a subject of ongoing debate. However, common features include intense and persistent emotions in both adults and children, such as overwhelming anger that isolates the individual and estranges the family, or complete suppression of any outward expression of emotion. Psychotherapy provides a secure and controlled environment for the expression of the grieving process. It has the potential to play a crucial role in the reconstruction, enhancement, and maintenance of the resources of both the individual and the family as they progress toward the future. The demands of dealing with bereavement necessitate mental health clinicians to possess a strong foundation in psychopathology, evaluation, and psychotherapy. Furthermore, a crucial aspect for professionals working with bereaved siblings is a deep understanding of child development and psychotherapy. In the absence of a comprehensive groundwork, healthcare professionals may find it challenging to contextualize the complex matters associated with grief, consequently impeding their efficacy in providing appropriate interventions. Providing support to families dealing with death and bereavement can be precarious territory for clinicians lacking experience or adequate support, regardless of their discipline. It is of utmost importance for clinicians to consistently monitor their own reactions and expressed beliefs during the process, refraining from passing judgment on how a family mourns. Seeking guidance from a colleague specializing in mental health can prove invaluable when navigating cri-

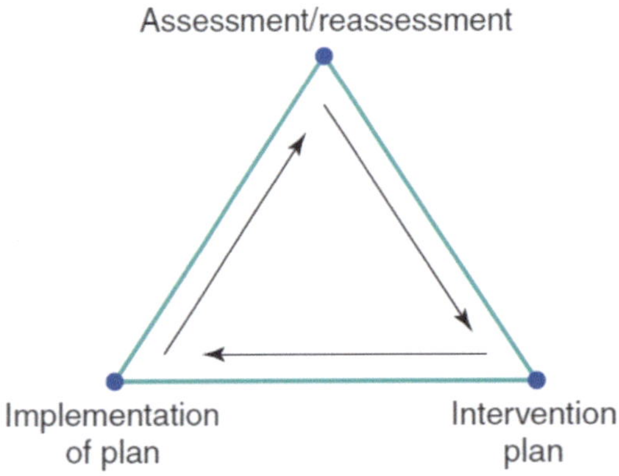


**Fig. 3.2** Assessment/intervention process. This figure is researcher-made design and has not been adapted from any resource

ses involving families. Furthermore, although many families may feel honored and touched by professionals expressing grief for their child, it is crucial for this compassion to be shown without overshadowing or surpassing the family's own emotional intensity. Clinicians have the ability to assess their level of involvement by considering the question: "Whose needs are being addressed?" Without any doubt, the correct answer is "The family's." This balanced perspective is an absolute of effective bereavement intervention. The impact of a child's death ripples through various spheres, from the immediate family to the wider community, encompassing the child's educational, residential, occupational, and religious environments. The child's death has profound impacts on these organizations, often requiring guidance to manage their shared grief. While it is not within the scope of palliative care clinicians to address all of these needs, they can significantly contribute by identifying and recommending appropriate care options [23]. Assessment/intervention process is provided in Fig. 3.2.

### 3.12.2 Useful Points for Bereavement Intervention

- Kindly allocate uninterrupted time to engage in conversation with the family, demonstrating your undivided attention.
- Ensure a comfortable and discreet physical environment, equipped with amenities such as tissues and water. When children are involved, make sure to provide toys, books, and supplies for drawing or writing.
- Extend a warm welcome to the family, convey your sympathies, and recognize the magnitude of their grief.
- It is advised to address the deceased child using their given name. Please consider the possibility of reviewing photographs of the child if they are provided by the family. Exercise discretion when considering initiating a request to view visual imagery.
- Approach the family in a manner that is open and nonjudgmental in order to foster trust and minimize any feeling of intimidation.
- Structure inquiries in a manner that aligns with the cognitive, developmental, and educational capacities, as well as the cultural heritage of the family.
- It is always advisable to ask rather than make assumptions.
- Before delving into the child's illness and demise, provide the family with an opportunity to recount and reflect on the child's life.
- Families are encouraged to narrate their child's story in a manner and timeframe of their preference. It is a common occurrence for those who have lost a loved one to frequently reiterate the details surrounding their illness and demise as they progress through the grieving process.
- Please proceed with the evaluation at a suitable pace. It is advised to refrain from overwhelming the family. Prioritizing speed during an interview in order to finish the assessment frequently leads to undue anxiety and the exclusion of vital details.
- Allow the family to freely articulate their emotions and viewpoints, irrespective of your concurrence. Kindly avoid interrupting or attempting to fill moments of silence.
- It is advisable to cross-reference your observations with the family. Whenever it is deemed necessary, make a point to explicitly inquire about the accuracy of your comprehension. In

the event that an error is made or a misunderstanding occurs, it is important to apologize and proceed. Forgiveness is often a characteristic found within families.
- In the event that warning signs arise during the evaluation, seek guidance from a mental health professional.
- Bereavement interviews evoke the expression of profound emotions. It is essential to closely observe your own responses during and following the session. In the same way that every family is unique, each clinician brings their own background and vulnerabilities to the setting [23].

## 3.13 Identifying Grief in a Child

Many children, especially younger children, experience symptoms of post-traumatic stress disorder (PTSD) after a traumatic event and bereavement, which include:

- Abdominal pains and headaches
- Sleep disorder (difficulty falling asleep or waking up)
- Irritability
- ADHD
- Anger
- Death game
- Asking repetitive questions
- Lack of self-confidence
- Relapse behaviors such as finger sucking or bedwetting
- Lack of positive emotions
- Persistent intense fear or sadness

## 3.14 Misconceptions about Children's Bereavement

- Children do not experience grief.

  It is not yet time to tell them.

- If the child does not talk about grief, neither should we.
- We must inform the child at an appropriate time.
- The child should not participate in the mourning ceremony.
- If we tell the child, his mind will be involved all the time.
- To protect the child, it is better not to tell him anything about death.

Whenever death is certain, we must tell the child.

## 3.15 Questions that May be Asked

- Can my child participate in the funeral ceremony?
- Should I tell my child the truth?
- How do I inform my other children about this?
- Will my child suffer psychological damage?
- How do I describe death to my child?
- My family members do not like young children to participate in ceremonies. What should I do?
- I don't think my child can handle this news. What do you think? [30].

## 3.16 Child's Participation in the Funeral Ceremony

- Participation in the ceremony is completely a personal decision of the family and depends on the interest of the child.
- If the child is interested in participating in the funeral, there is no prohibition.
- Participation in the funeral ceremony can help to understand the death and end of the person, but some children are not prepared for it. Never force a child to attend a funeral.
- If the child decides to attend the funeral, give him enough information about the ceremony and its events. Explain to the child that the funeral is a sad event and some people cry during it. If there is a casket or funeral, prepare the child for it.

- Explaining the mourning ceremony to the child and preparing him to participate in the ceremony does not mean that he should not be upset and express his sadness. The child can also become sad by participating in the ceremony, and his behavior is unpredictable.
- If you think that a funeral is not the best way for him to say goodbye to his lost loved one, use other methods. The teaching of death and termination of a relationship and separation.

## 3.17 Telling the Truth to the Child

- Many parents are faced with the issue of whether or not I should tell my child about the possibility of death.
- This issue depends on the family itself and considers the following factors:

  – Considering parents' wishes.
  – Attention to the child's condition.
  – Parents know their child.
  – Cultural, religious, and spiritual beliefs.
  – Child's questions.
  – Notifying other children of a family about the death of a sister/brother.
  – Involve your children in this subject according to their age.
  – Provide simple information about what is happening in plain language.
  – If your child is going to meet his/her sick sibling, thoroughly describe the changes your sick child will see before the visit, for example, "cutting his hair" or "currently he is unconscious and they are breathing through a tube" or "his hand is injured and he has a bandage."
  – Give your child a chance to say goodbye after meeting.
  – Talk to your children about what they expect from the ceremony and funeral after the death of their sibling.
  – Ask a friend or relative to be more with your child [54].

## 3.18 Children's Understanding and Reaction to Bereavement and Death at Different Ages

Grief reactions in children and young people will change over time and maturity and vary according to ss, culture, age, previous losses and experiences, family support, the relationship to the deceased, and the nature of the death.

Children's responses to death reflect the family's current culture, previous experiences, and their political and social environment. In fact, children's developmental differences in understanding the concept and reality of death affect the reaction to bereavement.

Infants and toddlers (1 month to 3 years old):

In fact, according to studies, how children imagine death before the formation of speech is not precisely known, because there is no way to evaluate the state of the idea of death in them. Children under the age of 3 do not understand much about death. Until the age of 2, they feel the loss, but they do not understand the meaning of death. Young children react by observing the crying, anger, or deprivation of their parents or siblings and in turn show symptoms of sadness such as sleepiness and sadness. In severe cases, they also show self-harm and mood disorders [54].

### 3.18.1 Infants' and Toddlers' Reactions to Death

- Return to previous level of behavior (showing less independence) like finger sucking.
- Separation anxiety.
- Change in routines is the biggest threat for toddlers with severe illness.
- Infants and toddlers understand that they are in dangerous situations by observing parents' behaviors such as depression, sadness, anger, and anxiety.
- Helping parents to cope with emotions, control emotions, and understand the needs of the child.

- Encouraging parents to attend the hospital and cooperate in the care plan increases the adaptation of the child and parents to a critical and potentially fatal disease [48].

### 3.18.2 Young Children (3 to 5 Years Old)

Because they are unable to understand the real cause, they cannot separate physical causes from psychological causes.

Magical thinking: They believe that this incident happened or this disease was caused due to their thinking.

The result of these thoughts in the child is a sense of responsibility for mistakes, punishment, and embarrassment.

At this age, they have usually heard the word death and have an implicit reference to it.

They consider them a kind of departure and probably a kind of sleep. In fact, they consider death to be a temporary issue and expect the person to return.

They may know the physical reality of death, but they cannot separate it from the ability to live. (For example, anyone who sleeps does not move, so death is the same.)

Because of their immature understanding of time, there is no real recognition of the universality and inevitability of death [23].

### 3.18.3 Young Children's Reaction to Death

- If minors get sick at this age, they think that this disease is a punishment for their thoughts and actions.
- Using therapeutic and diagnostic methods along with hospitalization can stabilize their beliefs about punishment.
- Sudden infant death syndrome (SIDS): It is one of the significant deaths that occur in healthy infants. If young children have siblings who suffer from this syndrome, they often blame themselves.
- Observing the signs of acute mourning of the parents by the child can be considered as a behavior to reject the child.
- When a child in the family gets sick, the parents' attention is taken away from the other children; it is natural that if there is a young child in the family, he blames the illness on the parents' lack of attention and changes.
- Young children feel the prolonged absence of parents from home more than older children; if they are told that their sick sibling will never come home, they may assume that the parent will never come home either. They don't come and their biggest fear is separation anxiety [38].

### 3.18.4 Reaction of School-Age Children (6 to 10 Years) Toward Death

Children at this age understand that death is permanent and there are various causes of death. They are curious to participate in funerals. They consider wrongdoings and bad thoughts to be related to death and feel guilty about the incidents. They are more logical than younger children, but they are not able to accurately interpret words and explanations. Therefore, it is necessary to question children's understanding of the described issues. Children at the age of 6–7 years imagine death as God and spirit or Satan, and the natural physiological explanation about death may be their mental preoccupation with death. At the age of 7 to 9 years, the child's understanding of death increases and becomes similar to adults. At this age, they understand the inevitability, irreversibility, and universality of death. At this age, they may ask many questions to understand the meaning of death. Children with incurable diseases and their siblings are more aware of death due to multiple visits to hospitals and treatment teams [11].

### 3.18.5 Teenagers' Reaction to Death

Due to being in the stage of acquiring identity, teenagers are not able to accept death as much as adults, although they understand the concept of death to the extent of adults, but they are still under the influence of magical thoughts and are exposed to feelings of guilt and shame. In order to take care of teenagers suffering from end-of-life diseases such as cancer, nurses must spend a lot of time with them. The questions of these teenagers should be given honest answers, and needs such as privacy should be respected [13].

## 3.19 The Experience of Bereavement in Children

A child who is at the end of life or who has lost a loved one should be taught that when someone dies, we can feel many things. Some of these are given below:

- Feeling guilty
- Confusion
- Anger and anger
- Embarrassment
- Worry
- Questions like why…?
- Meaninglessness

You must tell the child that:

- Crying can be a good thing because it allows us to vent our feelings.
- It is the same for all of us, children and adults, boys and girls, men and women.

So, if you see an adult crying, don't be upset; he will be fine.

Talking and crying together helps us feel less alone.

- We may feel angry or cry when someone dies and this does not make us a bad person.

Pay attention to these things:

- Talk about what happened in age-appropriate language and be honest and open, say, for example, man or death. Avoid expressions such as "fell asleep" or "fallen into eternal sleep," "passed away," or "passed away" because it will confuse him and make him afraid to sleep.
- Invite older children and teenagers to the conversation.
- Invite children to attend funerals and other religious ceremonies. If they are not allowed to participate, they feel left out.
- Maintain routine daily habits and care because children are very sensitive to daily routines. If you want some alone time, find an adult who will care for the child and who is not affected by the bereavement or levent.
- Tell children that it is okay to play, have fun, or be happy.
- Assist them in crafting a diary, memory box, or commemorative book to preserve the memory of the individual [47].

## 3.20 Grief Interventions

Three factors are considered in the evaluation of the bereaved child:

1. Individual factors such as school status, social support, and previous experiences with death.
2. Factors related to death such as being accidental or predictable and the relationship of the child with the deceased.
3. Culture, religion, and family norms about culture and religion: Family norms play an important role in how children express grief, and therapists and grief counselors should pay special attention to these factors [23].

### 3.20.1 Send a Letter to the Person Who Lost the Child

The things you need for this are a helium balloon and a paper and pencil. Ask the child to write a letter to someone who has lost and together with him attach the letter to the balloon. Release it in the sky and together with the child say goodbye balloons; this gives children a visual way to say goodbye to the person they've lost and also releases any guilt or anger they may have about it; this can happen on the child's birthday. Or that person and any situation where the child needs to talk to the person [54].

### 3.20.2 Using the Symbol and Metaphor of the Cloud

Ask the child to think it is a cloud and tell him:

- Think that you are a cloud that is very sad that the person he loved is no longer with him! Now kill that cloud!
- This exercise allows the child to use this symbol to express his emotions; for this exercise, watercolor and gouache and the use of finger paints are very suitable [44].

### 3.20.3 Box of Nostalgia

Ask the child to write his longings and unsaid words for the person he lost and put them in the longings box. Later you can go somewhere with the child and send them in the sky with balloons.

It is very important to take this period very seriously, and if needed, be sure to seek help from a good child psychologist [6].

### 3.20.4 Hints

Use specific situations to teach death. For many children, the death of a pet is the first experience of death, and do not try to quickly replace another animal and do not make this event less important. Give the child time to grieve.

The death of a grandparent is another experience for children, and they ask you many questions. For example, they ask, "Is mother going to die soon?" You must tell your child that his mother will live with him for a long time.

After the death of one parent, children become extremely worried about the death of the other parent or other caregivers. Reassure the child that you will always love him and take care of him.

### 3.20.5 Do Not Neglect Parent Mourning

Children usually imitate their parents' behavior patterns; by showing your sadness, show him that you are sad and accept his sadness. Your extreme and uncontrollable behavior teaches the child unhealthy ways to deal with grief.

### 3.20.6 Describe Life after Death to a Child

It will be helpful for the bereaved child to describe life after death. If your religious beliefs believe in life after death, explain them to the child. But if you are not religious and do not believe in life after death, you can tell the child that the deceased will live on in the hearts and memories of the surviving loved ones. You can make a scrapbook or plant a plant that represents the person who was lost [55].

# 4 Spiritual Care

## 4.1 Spiritual Care Definition

One of the key focuses of palliative care services is addressing and fulfilling the spiritual and religious requirements of patients, particularly those with incurable conditions. Spiritual needs surpass the scope of religious needs. The inclusion of spiritual care is essential in order to support patients and families in their quest for meaning and purpose, as well as facilitating continued connection and personal transcendence. The identification and acknowledgment of the spiritual dimension in individuals is a fundamental element of caregiving, with spirituality being a key focus within the realm of nursing. The provision of spiritual care has a profound effect on the inner being of another individual [5].

Spirituality encompasses the perception of being linked to a greater entity and usually involves a pursuit for significance and purpose in life. People have the potential to designate a spiritual occurrence as sacred or transcendent or to encounter a profound sensation of liveliness and interconnectedness. The spiritual lives of certain individuals are intertwined with a religious organization, such as a church, temple, mosque, or synagogue. Conversely, some find solace and derive comfort from a personal connection to God or a higher power. Furthermore, others discover purpose through their bonds with nature or artistic endeavors. The perception of spirituality and sense of purpose in an individual often undergo alterations throughout their lifetime, influenced by personal experiences and relationships [56].

Examples of spiritual care: This care can be shared laughter or tears or staying awake with a family member whose loved one is struggling to recover from an illness. It can be crying with the patient's family when their patient dies. It can be taking care of and comforting a person affected by a chronic disease who is sitting somewhere. It may be a conversation at 3 o'clock in the morning before a surgery, or it may be accompanying in prayer or reading the Bible, the Quran, or other religious books that have a special meaning for the patient.

Many people who get cancer and even their families are involved in questions like "Why do I/my child have cancer?" or "Where has God's justice gone?" Or they experience despair and even suicidal thoughts. The main reason for these behaviors is the sense of emptiness and impasse of patients/families.

"Spiritual caregiver" accompanies the patient and those around him in various philosophical, spiritual, religious, and moral challenges such as right and wrong, reward and sin, justice, prayer and response, trust, patience, satisfaction, wisdom, hope, spiritual peace, self-esteem, self-awareness, knowledge of God, integration with nature and God-centered nature, fear of death, mourning, attention to oneself, interpersonal relationships, and even Sharia rules. Spiritual


N. Javadi-Pashaki et al., *Interdisciplinary Pediatric Palliative Care*,
https://doi.org/10.1007/978-981-97-9587-1_4

care services are provided in the form of individual counseling and spiritual group therapy sessions, and they help people to find the meaning of life again or to get a meaningful interpretation of the difficult experiences they are going through.

Spiritual care for cancer patients should be provided by an interdisciplinary team, but because nurses have the most contact with patients, they can take effective measures in this direction to increase the quality of their care. Unfortunately, due to lack of time, lack of manpower, and lack of sufficient training, this aspect of care for cancer patients is often neglected. It is necessary to form a team to provide spiritual care consisting of doctor, nurse, social worker, psychologist, and clergy in the hospital.

## 4.2 Distinguishing "Religion" from "Spirituality"

In its definition of palliative care, the WHO emphasized the importance of early identification, thorough assessment, and effective treatment of pain and other physical, psychosocial, and spiritual problems, with the goal of "preventing and relieving suffering" [57]. The notion that the care of the spirit is exclusively within the domain of religious leaders or chaplains arises from a lack of discernment between spirituality and religion among PC practitioners. While meaning and connectedness form the foundation of both religion and spirituality, religion is frequently characterized as the external embodiment of these principles, contrasting with spirituality that encompasses the internal encounter [58]. Emile Durkheim's definition of religion encompasses "the collective respect for the supernatural, sacred, or spiritual, as well as the symbols, rituals, and worship connected to it" [59]. He assigned designations to religions such as Christianity, Judaism, Hinduism, Islam, and Buddhism, acknowledging their divergent viewpoints, organizational structures, guidelines, and observances for their adherents. Nonetheless, spirituality is a considerably broader notion, encompassing the very core of human existence, and is perceived as that which bestows significance, direction, and interconnectivity to each distinct individual, regardless of their age. It is possible for a child to articulate their spirituality within the context of a religious framework, as exemplified by Ming, or they may possess a myriad of experiences and thoughts that extend beyond conventional religious practices, thereby engendering significance. It is possible for religion and spirituality to have a connection in the case of some individuals. Within the realm of CPC, it is crucial that we grasp these concepts and constructs not only for the child but also for their siblings, parents, and other individuals who play a supportive role in their life. While there are various definitions of spirituality, one commonly accepted consensus definition that has been developed from the National Consensus Project earlier definitions is one that we propose can be used practically in CPC: "Spirituality is a dynamic and intrinsic aspect of humanity through which persons seek ultimate meaning, purpose and transcendence, and experience relationship to self, family, others, community, society, nature and the significant or sacred. Spirituality is expressed through beliefs, values, traditions and practices" [60, 61]. Spirituality entails the child's search for meaning resulting from their experiences and questions such as "Who am I?", "What does my life mean?", and "What is happening to me and my family?". The child and family may not necessarily seek definitive responses to these existential queries, but rather seek solace, hope, and a sense of security in order to ask them. At the core of spirituality and the quest for significance resides mystery and paradox.

## 4.3 The Process and Stages of Spiritual Care

1. In this stage, the nurse performs a purposeful assessment of the patient's condition, with the intention of investigating and recognizing spiritual perspectives (Fig. 4.1).

(A) **Spiritual Screening:** To assess, a series of straightforward questions are posed: "To what extent does religion and spirituality

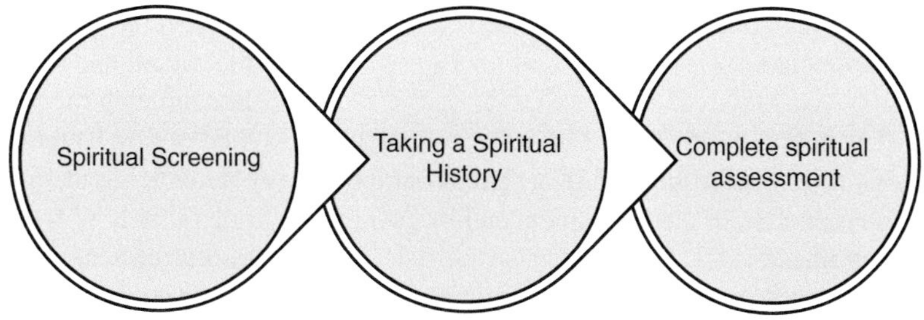


**Fig. 4.1** Assessment/intervention process. This figure is researcher-made design and has not been adapted from any resource

play a significant role in your adaptation?". Should the patient/family emphasize the significance of spirituality? An additional query could be posed, "To what extent are these resources meeting your needs?" When the patient communicates difficulties with adjustment and/or indicates insufficient efficacy of spiritual or religious resources, a comprehensive evaluation and referral to a spiritual care professional is warranted.

(B) **Conducting a Spiritual History:** A spiritual history involves a series of questions aimed at encouraging patients and their family members to explore their spiritual and religious beliefs as well as their needs in this regard. The inclusion of a spiritual history holds particular significance during the initial consultation.

Currently, the aim is to gain a deeper understanding of the patient's beliefs and values.

(C) **Comprehensive Spiritual Evaluation:** If the nurse deems it necessary for the patient to engage in a more extensive conversation with a specialist in spiritual care, it is advisable to conduct a formal spiritual assessment. The objective is to comprehend the requirements and available resources in the patient's family through attentive listening to the patient's narrative. The nurse should conduct a thorough assessment of the patient, including inquiries about topics such as meaning, purpose, and hope; their relationship with God; spiritual practices; religious commitments; interpersonal communication; and the professional interactions of the staff [62, 63].

**In the field of spirituality, there exist several nursing diagnoses, including:**

Spiritual distress: This refers to the condition of anguish and torment caused by the hindered capacity to find significance in life through self-reflection, interpersonal connections, the natural world, or a higher power.

Religiosity disorder: This is characterized by the impaired capacity to rely on religious beliefs or engage in specific traditional religious ceremonies.

The inclination to enhance religiosity: It is the readiness or capacity to augment dependence on religious beliefs or engage in community-specific religious rituals.

## 4.4 Planning and Implementation of Spiritual Care

Once the nurse, in collaboration with the patient, identifies their needs, concerns, and spiritual strengths, it becomes imperative to develop a comprehensive plan that addresses these aspects. This program includes identifying the goals of spiritual care and determining spiritual care activities.

Purposes of Spiritual Care

1. The alleviation of suffering and discomfort and the capacity to derive existential meaning through self-reflection, interpersonal interaction, engagement with the world, or connection with a higher power.
2. Expressing the feeling of satisfaction and peace in the context of communication with a creator.
3. Having a pleasant feeling about life.
4. Having hope in life and trusting in God.

Spiritual care activities and interventions for nurses include:

- Creating a positive mindset in the patient and family from the moment of arrival through the introduction of the department and its governing rules.
- Quick response to calling the patient/patient's companion and addressing the patient's needs at the moment of care and relieving the patient's symptoms.
- Providing sufficient and understandable explanations to the patient and family in relation to care and treatment measures.
- Valuing patients and families at any level of economic, social, or ethnic status.
- Setting aside external factors and focusing willfully on work in order to have real presence.
- Having a regular shift schedule for active and therapeutic presence at the patient's bedside.
- Showing love, kindness, and compassion during care (talking more with the patient and family while providing care, such as administering medications).
- Empathy and sympathy with the patient in order to show compassionate and altruistic presence.
- Listening actively and deeply to the patient's stories and facilitating the expression of these stories to help the patient achieve meaning.
- Not judging the patient and not imposing his views and opinions on the patient.
- Using appropriate communication skills such as asking and active listening and using silence where appropriate.
- Paying attention to the patient's verbal and non-verbal signs such as eye contact, tone of voice, and appearance that indicates a spiritual concern.
- Supporting and showing ethical behavior while communicating with the patient, such as being honest and polite, respecting people regardless of religious beliefs, and being loyal.
- Understanding the patient's condition and identifying oneself with the patient in order to respond appropriately to the patient's emotions and feelings.
- Respecting the dignity, values, and beliefs of the patient and family.
- Encouraging the patient to communicate with God or a higher power such as praying to God.
- Encouraging the patient to communicate with others such as friends and family, especially during critical moments such as using telephone communication when needed.
- Encouraging the patient to communicate with nature, such as walking in the green space.
- Helping the patient to feel hopeful by identifying the positive aspects of the patient.
- Encouraging the patient to perform religious activities if desired and facilitating the spiritual concerns of the patient through prayer.
- Preservation of patient privacy during care and treatment.
- Trying to remain confidential and keep the secrets of the patient.
- Trying to create a safe and relaxing treatment environment in order to make the patient feel comfortable by taking measures such as creating a positive mindset when admitted to the hospital, improving work relationships with colleagues, supporting colleagues, creating a pleasant working environment for themselves and patients, avoiding excesses, and understanding needs.
- Investigating the effectiveness of spiritual care with the patient by encouraging the patient to express his spiritual state after care and discussing the results with the patient and recording them based on the appropriate pattern.
- Recording spiritual care interventions and their results in the patient's care file.

In hospitalized children, listening empathetically and talking about the spiritual journey is the most effective spiritual intervention to meet their needs.

## 4.5 Evaluation and Documentation

Engaging in a conversation with the patient stands as the most evident approach to assess the efficacy of spiritual care. In this particular context, signs that indicate a sense of well-being, assurance in receiving care, and absence of concerns about both care and the present circumstances can be beneficial. Upon finishing the provision of spiritual care, it is the nurse's duty to carry out documentation. The recorded data in this stage encompasses the patient's pre-intervention condition, the intervention carried out, the patient's response, and the outcomes.

## 4.6 Patient Scenario

Mr. Yun, a 14-year-old boy, has come to his physician's office to report difficulties with concentration, feelings of sadness, and symptoms of anxiety. The patient has recently suffered the loss of his mother in a motor vehicle accident and is currently experiencing insomnia and a significant weight loss of over 15 pounds within the past month. He articulates feelings of despair and resentment toward God due to the loss he has encountered. He affirms that he used to participate in religious services with his mother, although he emphasizes that it was primarily her preference. I really don't know "what to believe anymore."

### 4.6.1 Applying the Nursing Process

**Assessment:** Findings indicate that the patient is encountering challenges in maintaining focus, experiencing emotions of sadness and hopelessness, and reporting symptoms of anxiety. He expresses feelings of despair, anger toward God, and doubts in his belief system through self-reporting.

A nursing care plan has been formulated for Mr. Yun, taking into account the assessment information that has been collected.

**Nursing Diagnosis:** The nursing diagnosis of spiritual distress is present, stemming from the loss of a challenged belief system. This is evident through self-reported feelings of "hopelessness," being "angry at God," and a general sense of uncertainty in beliefs.

**Overall Goal:** The objective is for the patient to exhibit enhanced spirituality.

**SMART Expected Outcome:** As the teaching session draws to a close, Mr. Yun will describe a spiritual practice that brings him comfort.

### 4.6.2 Planning and Implementing Nursing Interventions

The nurse will determine the factors that impact the patient's personal belief system. The nurse will offer assistance to the patient, enabling them to express their emotions and anger. The nurse will engage in empathetic observation and attentive listening during the communication process. The nurse will actively encourage the utilization of spiritual resources and request the patient's authorization to initiate contact with a chaplain.

### 4.6.3 Sample Documentation

Mr. Yun demonstrates indications of spiritual distress following the demise of his mother, which has caused a disruption in his personal belief system. He expresses feelings of anger, hopelessness, and uncertainty within his belief system. Nonetheless, he discovers solace by immersing himself in the great outdoors. The patient's consent has been obtained to engage a chaplain in order to attend to Mr. Yun's spiritual requirements.

### 4.6.4 Evaluation

Following the conclusion of the teaching session, the nurse informs Mr. Yun that a chaplain will contact him at his residence, with his consent, for further communication. Permission for the referral has been granted by Mr. Yun. The nurse inquires about the additional spiritual resources Mr. Yun intends to utilize in his home. Mr. Yun states his intention to deliberately partake in daily outdoor walks for the purpose of immersing himself in nature. The SMART objective was successfully achieved [56].

# 5 Teamwork

## 5.1 Interdisciplinary Team

The inclusion of interdisciplinary teams is a widespread practice in numerous palliative care settings globally. Many experts regard teamwork as an essential function of palliative care teams. The notable variations in structure and function of these teams within regional and organizational contexts have the potential to influence both their strengths and weaknesses in terms of overall productivity. The team's sustainability and resilience indirectly impact its functioning. An interdisciplinary team requires the inclusion of diverse disciplines [64] (Fig. 5.1).

## 5.2 Enhancing Team Development

In order for a group of individuals to transform into a cohesive team, they must collectively embrace a shared objective, exhibit unwavering dedication toward accomplishing specific objectives, and prioritize the significance of collabora-

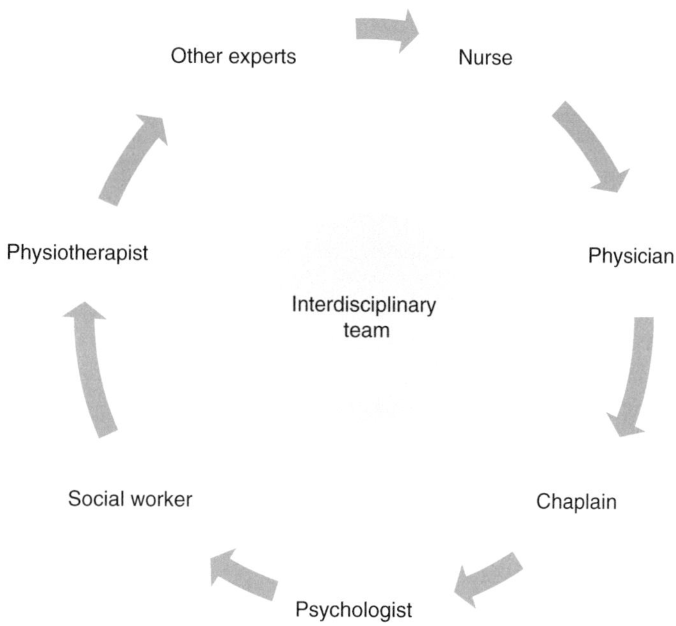


**Fig. 5.1** Different profession in an interdisciplinary team. This figure is researcher-made design and has not been adapted from any resource


N. Javadi-Pashaki et al., *Interdisciplinary Pediatric Palliative Care*,
https://doi.org/10.1007/978-981-97-9587-1_5

tive efforts to yield greater outcomes. The transition from a group to a team is facilitated by establishing individual ownership of clearly defined tasks and ensuring the sharing of outcomes [65].

Size and leadership are additional distinguishing factors between groups and teams. Although the size of groups may differ, teams consist of only a small number of members who jointly assume leadership responsibilities in clinical practice. However, at an administrative level, they are guided by a senior member. Depending on the child's condition and the family's circumstances, various professionals may assume leadership roles at different times, making unique contributions to accomplish the team's objectives and tasks.

Irrespective of whether a team opts for a manager to facilitate action coordination or embraces self-management, it is crucial to ensure shared responsibility for outcomes. In contrast, within a group setting, leadership is typically delegated to a single individual who enforces their leadership style, which often remains unaltered regardless of shifts in focus or work tasks [66].

Our perspective regards teams as dynamic systems capable of development, expansion, and operating with higher levels of transparency, communication, and cooperation among caregivers. The development of a team does not follow a linear trajectory. It is defined by alternating cycles of progressive and regressive motion, as well as intervals of stability, disorganization, stagnation, and development. The level of development of a team is determined by the members' ability to establish and maintain collaborations that provide quality care and enrichment to both families and team members. Among the various models for comprehending team development, particularly in the context of palliative care, the ones proposed by Papadatou and Morasz are noteworthy. They maintain the viewpoint that throughout the development process, team members undergo phases of coexistence, mutual recognition, and parallel collaboration, as well as collaborative alliances resulting in changes to disciplinary boundaries [67, 68].

When operating within the realm of coexistence, professionals tend to collaborate more as a collective rather than as a cohesive team. Typically, goals are shared, specific roles are assigned, and tasks are distributed among care providers who deliver fragmented and compartmentalized services. Families of seriously ill children are often provided with a predetermined package of medical, nursing, psychological, social, and spiritual services. Subsequently, they are introduced or referred to various experts.

Transactions within professional circles often exhibit inflexibility and limited communication. Infrequently do they provide their colleagues with reports on the nature and outcomes of their intervention or observations, despite the potential usefulness of such information in their interactions with families. Every care provider concentrates on their specific area of expertise and conveys their accomplishments through concise reports typically documented in the patient's file. Care providers initiate collaborative efforts by adopting a mode of parallel collaboration. They mutually recognize each other's expertise and abilities and collaborate in parallel yet autonomous manners to achieve common objectives and assignments. The transactions have become more comprehensive, and the communication has become more transparent, yet it still lacks depth. The team members successfully complete their tasks, yet they are unable to incorporate the full range of existing services into a coherent and comprehensive framework.

In the context of parallel collaboration, teamwork typically involves multiple disciplines, with team members not necessarily adjusting their roles and responsibilities to align with those of other professionals. Typically, information is conveyed through the patient's file or during staff meetings, where each provider presents their work without fully integrating it into the care plan provided to the child and family. Effective and open communication is prioritized in the collaborative alliance among professionals engaged in planning, offering, and evaluating their collective services. Information is circulated among team members, fostering a culture of learning where individuals broaden their horizons, critically analyze their work, and acknowledge their strengths and limitations. Their collaboration emphasizes the importance of a reflective process, with periodic evaluations of outcomes and service provision methods to ensure goal attainment.

Teamwork has transitioned into an interdisciplinary practice that relies on the close cooperation of professionals who establish specific goals, deliberate on strategies, and collectively assume responsibility for the care, rather than acting as individuals.

Team members exhibit a strong sense of interconnectedness and belonging. The prioritization of team identity supersedes individual identities. The establishment of mutual support is crucial when working toward collective objectives and addressing the inherent challenges and difficulties in caregiving. The distribution of leadership, responsibility, and accountability is typically shared among interdisciplinary teams.

Within proficient and harmonious teams, collaboration often manifests as a transdisciplinary partnership. Care providers engage in mutual training in specific areas of their expertise to expand their knowledge and skills, enabling them to effectively address diverse needs without unnecessary duplication of services. This aspect becomes particularly crucial when it comes to the care of terminally ill children, especially in cases where families opt to restrict their engagement with professionals and instead concentrate on the child's well-being and their own. To establish a collaborative alliance, care providers must dedicate time to working collectively, exchanging experiences, examining various perspectives, and cultivating an inclusive shared language. In order for interdisciplinary and transdisciplinary teamwork to be successful, the team must collaborate interdependently and operate as an open system that incorporates relevant information. Information that is pertinent includes data that enables members to grasp their systemic functioning, navigate through suffering and adversities, and optimize resource utilization [67]. The provision of such information enables team members to learn from experience, explore alternative ideas and coping patterns, embrace new initiatives, take calculated risks, implement changes, and foster team growth. In the absence of the chance to exchange information on daily work, task execution, and professional attitudes, team members are unable to maintain control over the quality of their services, resulting in an uncorrectable system [69]. This level of openness goes beyond merely expressing emotions and thoughts. It necessitates a reflective mindset that empowers team members to question their own and others' thoughts, embrace ambiguity, and share experiences with a willingness to have them scrutinized or modified [68, 70].

In a team of this nature, care providers find satisfaction in delivering services that are both beneficial and significant to patients and families while also engaging in collaborative endeavors to achieve a common goal.

## 5.3 Models for Teamwork

The team's structure and member interactions differ depending on the teamwork model. In an Australian context, Crawford and Price (2003) have outlined three models of healthcare teams. In the scenario of a purely multidisciplinary team, individuals are assigned clearly defined responsibilities. Rather than engaging with fellow team members, each professional delivers care independently. This approach is widely recognized to possess practical limitations, primarily stemming from the fragmentation of care. On the opposite end of the spectrum lies the transdisciplinary approach, characterized by a greater extent of overlapping responsibilities among its members [71]. Each member is expected to fulfill identical responsibilities throughout their shift. The presence of unmet specific care needs makes this model generally unsuitable for healthcare teams. Within an interdisciplinary team, members engage in mutual interaction and interdependent collaboration, ultimately enhancing the delivery of comprehensive patient care. This model is particularly well-suited for palliative care provision [64].

The members of the multidisciplinary team in palliative care encompass doctors, nurses, and allied health professionals (AHPs). The care team consists of various physicians, such as general practitioners, palliative physicians, psychiatrists, oncologists, and specialists in specific diseases, like nephrologists [72]. Nurse practitioners and community nurses have a significant impact, as do AHPs [73]. AHP encompasses various healthcare professionals, including physiotherapists, occupational therapists, speech and language therapists, dietitians, and numerous other therapists [72]. Patients receive assistance in their psychosocial well-being from professionals such as psychologists, counselors, social workers, and community volunteers, while spiritual guidance is provided by priests, chaplains, and pastoral caregivers [74]. The permanent members of a team, known as the core team, are comprised of individuals whose services are crucial and are needed regularly. The extended team is composed of individuals who offer support as required [75]. In addition, extended team members play a vital role in providing essential aspects of care. This may encompass solicitors who offer assistance to patients in advanced care planning, such as appointing lasting power of attorney for welfare and financial matters [76]. Family members and caregivers, who play a crucial role in providing care, are also considered part of the team [77], especially in countries with established palliative care systems like the United Kingdom and Australia. The skill sets of team members can exhibit substantial variations across countries and regions, influenced by locoregional needs, policies, and resources. As an illustration, volunteers have been a long-standing component of the hospice workforce in the United Kingdom [71]. However, they are deployed in broader community-based capacities in other regions with less well-equipped palliative care systems, like Kerala, India [78].

### 5.3.1 Phases of Team Development

The growth of a team evolves through successive stages, during which the members develop and acquire experience [78]. During the initial "forming" stage, inexperienced members make an effort to establish their roles under the supervision of a designated leader. Conflicts arise in the "storming" stage due to conflicting opinions within subgroups and a desire for power. The phase known as "norming" entails members reconciling with their designated roles and duties. They engage in open discussions about their concerns with fellow members who they have a deep sense of belonging with. During the concluding phase of "performing," team members collaborate to achieve synergy and establish internal conflict resolution mechanisms [79]. The concept of a "phases model" posits that a team does not initially operate efficiently, but rather achieves efficiency by developing as a cohesive group.

Among the various teamwork philosophies (directive, integrative, elective), the integrative model is widely regarded as the most effective for palliative care MDTs. The value attributed to each professional in this model is considered equal as their combined expertise allows for the holistic care of patients. The group's functioning relies on frequent discussions among its members. A leadership approach that is more directive is implemented to identify the skill sets of team players, allocate appropriate tasks, inspire, cooperate with external resources, handle obstacles, and guide the overall performance of the team toward the accomplishment of established objectives. When directive leadership effectively coordinates the roles and responsibilities of team players, it is probable that patients, practitioners, and caregivers will all experience positive outcomes. When there is a lack of supportive leadership, teamwork can be an exasperating endeavor. The team's functioning can be compromised by a deficient understanding of leadership and disputes regarding authority. From time to time, teams may confront challenges associated with members who display undue dominance [80]. The gold standard framework has played a crucial role in connecting communication with the delivery of high-quality generalist palliative care, in which well-coordinated teams have utilized a combination of formal and informal gatherings [81]. The intention was for the meetings to be conducted in a non-hierarchical manner, with minimal emphasis on leadership. However, the doctor-nurse relationship did reveal a certain degree of hierarchy. According to a qualitative study carried out in Sweden, the importance of communication was emphasized as essential for the delivery of palliative care and the effective functioning of teams. Effective interprofessional communication is considered crucial for making management decisions, resolving conflicts, establishing trust, fulfilling administrative duties, advocating for others, sharing knowledge and experiences, and ultimately improving individual and collective competencies [82]. According to a study conducted in Switzerland, the absence of formal communication channels among professionals in various care settings has resulted in disharmony [83]. Healthcare professionals encounter various communication obstacles when interacting with patients diagnosed with life-threatening illnesses, such as delivering unfavorable news, handling collusion, addressing difficult inquiries, managing uncertainty, and responding to overt emotional responses [84]. The preferred team member for a patient can vary depending on the individual [85]. This concept suggests that the presence of team members with diverse personality traits can be seen as a source of strength. Team members possessing extensive expertise in leadership, communication skills, trust-building, and team development are suitably equipped to function as adept intermediaries in managing dissonance. Furthermore, they are capable of providing invaluable feedback and support to their colleagues [86]. The composition of the conventional palliative care team is undergoing ongoing changes. Within the Taiwanese context, there are examples of music and art therapists who offer services that mitigate symptoms and promote an enhanced quality of life for patients [87]. The apprehension regarding negative consequences of drug treatment, such as opiophobia, may contribute to patients' hesitancy in embracing pharmacotherapy. Patients receiving care in resource-rich settings, where a variety of therapeutic approaches are available, offer potential for investigating the benefits of complementary therapies, including art therapy. As a result of inherent disparities in the training, exposure, and perspectives of the diverse professionals engaged, it is expected that contrasting viewpoints regarding the most suitable therapeutic modality for a patient based on their current status will emerge. Silbermann et al.'s findings indicate the possibility of interprofessional conflict [88]. Multidisciplinary team (MDT) discussions provide an opportunity for team members to carefully consider each option and reach a consensus on the most optimal management plan for a patient. Care decisions within palliative care are made with a strong emphasis on respecting a patient-centered approach [89]. The overlap in role designations among distinct personnel implies their primary function within the team. In reality, though, there will likely be a substantial overlap between roles. To provide an example, hospice chaplains who embrace a multi-faith perspective can offer spiritual guidance to patients regardless of their religious background or spiritual beliefs. Dutch experts suggest that other team members, not principally concerned with spiritual care provision, should also have a basic training in assessing spiritual distress and an overview of the nature of care a pastoral caregiver provides [90]. This level of comprehension guarantees that healthcare professionals are more likely to recognize spiritual distress and take appropriate measures, including making appropriate referrals, to alleviate it. It is not unusual for dissonance to arise when there is uncertainty regarding the specific roles of individual professionals. Disagreements can occur among professionals who claim sole responsibility for a particular aspect of a person's medical care. Instances may arise where professionals inadvertently neglect certain aspects of care due to the assumption that another colleague is responsible [91]. Ensuring prompt communication among team members can help prevent such incidents.

### 5.3.2 Dealing with Burnout and Compassion Fatigue

Palliative care providers are responsible for managing emotionally and occasionally physically overwhelming tasks, as they navigate the challenges of supporting individuals facing mortality, suffering, and uncertainty, which can leave them susceptible to compassion fatigue and burnout. The occurrence of burnout encompasses mental, emotional, and physical fatigue, which can potentially diminish a professional's motivation and competence. In hospice and palliative care settings, the prevalence of burnout among clinicians, primarily attributed to emotional exhaustion, can reach as high as 62%. Recent research has indicated that conflicts within a team can be a significant cause of stress. Nevertheless, collaboration within a team has the potential to positively impact individuals by strengthening interpersonal connections, facilitating professional evaluation, and fostering the exchange of experiences, responsibilities, and concerns [92].

## 5.4 Organizational Culture and Context

The progress of a team is not solely contingent upon the individuals within it [67, 93]. The development and functioning of a service are greatly influenced by the social and organizational context in which it operates. As an illustration, in certain regions, pediatric palliative care services are provided by community-based teams through home, respite, or hospice programs. Furthermore, they are introduced within the confines of the hospital and extend consultation services to professionals, families, and other teams. In numerous countries with limited resources or a reluctance to address the requirements of terminally ill children and mourning families, the availability of palliative care teams is either absent or hindered by significant social, institutional, and legal challenges. In nations with abundant resources that recognize the importance of supporting terminally ill children and their mourning families, the delivery of interdisciplinary and palliative care services may face obstacles due to the structure of the healthcare system. The cultural norms within a social context shape the organizational culture and services of a team, thus exerting an influence on the services offered. The role of the organization's culture is significant in shaping the perception, care, and integration of seriously ill children within the organization or service. When a child's life is at stake, organizational culture plays a role in regulating suffering, instilling hope, and managing time. Certain organizations that adopt a cure-oriented approach often disregard or minimize the importance of palliative care services. Instead, they opt for a protective approach by concealing the notion of death from both the child and occasionally the parents. Several organizations strive to integrate curative, life-prolonging, and palliative care services, promoting collaboration among multiple teams and involved family members in the decision-making process. As a result, the dynamics of teamwork within an organization or service can be influenced, either positively or negatively, by its care philosophy, values, goals, and priorities. It is important to note that teams still have the ability to shape their own development. However, certain teams receive support and guidance throughout this process, while others face the challenge of independently establishing and advancing their approach within the healthcare system.

## 5.5 Teams at Work

### 5.5.1 Indicators of Team Development, Functionality, and Effectiveness

We firmly believe that teams possess the potential to change, develop, and thrive. Teams, similar to the individuals comprising them, are not passive actors. Teams, similar to their members, act as active agents who mutually influence and are influenced by their individual and collective reactions to life-threatening diseases, grief, distress, and the individuals they engage with in their profession. Teams, similar to their members, experience and respond to various internal and external stressors associated with the management of seriously ill patients and their families. In light of the broader social and organizational work environment, team members make deliberate or subconscious choices regarding their operational and collaborative approaches, aiming to overcome life-or-death challenges. The team's ability to develop, function, and be effective is demonstrated through the patterns in which its members navigate team boundaries, manage team operations, and deal with challenges and time constraints [67].

#### 5.5.1.1 Team Boundaries

Teams characterized by well-defined yet adaptable and permeable boundaries are conducive to interdisciplinary collaborations and foster a culture of open teamwork. In contrast, teams with rigid boundaries tend to function as closed systems in which transactions are tightly controlled and collaboration is limited. Similarly, teams characterized by diffused or blurred boundaries subject their members to intrusions and invasions from both internal and external sources, resulting in chaotic transactions that perpetuate constant distress within intra- and inter-team relationships. Their development is compromised as they become excessively engrossed in their conflicts rather than embracing opportunities for learning, collaborating, and growth.

#### 5.5.1.2 Team Operation

Organizations that establish explicit and achievable objectives, supported by a comprehensive and integrated care strategy, facilitate transparent communication and collaborative partnership that yield advantages for both families and professionals. Within these teams, healthcare providers establish a method of operation that is regularly assessed and adjusted to accommodate evolving situations and emerging needs. Rather than being avoided, losses, traumas, and achievements are openly acknowledged, and team resources are effectively leveraged to handle crises or challenging situations. In contrast, teams that have unclear or unrealistic goals, as well as blurred roles and functions, often distribute accountability among members who compartmentalize their services and work autonomously. The lack of cooperation in crisis or traumatic event management leads to its suppression, concealment, or implementation. The team's functioning is rarely assessed, resulting in the formation and perpetuation of dysfunctional patterns.

#### 5.5.1.3 Management of Suffering

Teams serve as repositories for the suffering experienced by both children, families, and their own members. When team members acknowledge and confront the suffering caused by the threat to a child's life, they are able to integrate painful experiences into their daily functioning without becoming incapacitated or overwhelmed by them. Recognizing and acknowledging suffering serves as a driving force for them to create a secure environment where families and team members can openly express, explore, accept, and ultimately overcome their suffering. On the other hand, teams that make efforts to eradicate, conceal, or repress suffering, viewing it as an indication of vulnerability and inadequacy, are prone to forming detached or entangled relationships that undermine substantial partnerships with children, families, and colleagues, thus impeding the team's growth.

#### 5.5.1.4 Experience and Management of Time

When a child's life is endangered by a severe condition, families and care providers perceive and experience time in distinct manners [94]. A team that prioritizes their work fosters an environment where children and their families can contemplate and navigate their grief while also embracing a purposeful existence. Moreover, the team understands the importance of addressing work-related experiences that elicit anxiety among team members. The team acquires wisdom from previous experiences, incorporates that knowledge into present practices, and endeavors to achieve future objectives focused on improving the quality of the services it delivers. On the other hand, teams that refrain from addressing difficult subjects and experiences become stagnant. The ability of these teams to take action, make decisions, and enact interventions becomes impaired. They delve deeply into the realms of apathy and inertia. They enter a state of temporal stasis. There are teams that exhibit a behavior suggesting the elimination of time. Their workload is overwhelmingly high. The experience of time is marked by the occurrence of various events. Events or crises serve as the driving force behind work. The continuous state of excessive agitation hinders the team from taking a pause to reflect on their experiences and utilize pertinent information for the purpose of learning, evolving, and developing [67].

## 5.6 Teams and Families

### 5.6.1 A Partnership in Care

A significant number of parents aim to take on a central and proactive role in the caregiving of their child who is experiencing illness. They gain extensive knowledge of the child's condition and treatments and acquire the necessary skills to meet their intricate needs. Parents of critically ill children encounter unique challenges and crises that surpass any previous experience in their lives [95]. To ensure their effectiveness in this new parenting role, they must engage with professionals who can assist them in developing strategies and skills to handle current situations and anticipate future needs for their sick and healthy children. The frequent engagement can often result in the mistaken belief that parents are part of the team. In contrast to certain clinicians who have written on the subject of teams and palliative care, we hold the stance that parents and patients do not qualify as team members. Referring to a patient or parent as a team member is most effective at a metaphorical level, although even then, it can be misleading. It is not possible for a parent or child to fully participate as a member of a multidisciplinary or interdisciplinary team. The team's rich history, encompassing both triumphs and challenges, is not acknowledged or recognized by them. Furthermore, their goals, values, and priorities may not align with those of the team and the families it serves. Furthermore, regarding parents and patients as team members diminishes the distinctive bond that exists between sick children and their parents, as well as between teams and the individuals they assist. A more suitable manner of conceptualizing the position of the patient and parents in relation to the team is to perceive them as occupying a symbolic realm where care is both provided and received. The ownership of this space does not pertain to either the family or the team, but rather to their distinct relationship. The hope is that the relationship will progress and transform into a partnership. As partners, professionals and families collaborate to establish care objectives, which may evolve throughout the progression of the illness, and depend on one another to accomplish them. While team members are tasked with the responsibility of offering information, guidance, advice, and specialized care, family members are expected to actively engage in decision-making processes and effectively communicate their needs, concerns, values, and preferences. When creating a care plan, it is important to consider the family's obligations.

When dealing with this partnership, it is imperative to give careful consideration and handle with expertise the views, concerns, and desires of children. It is essential to be mindful of the disparities in how children communicate their physical, psychosocial, and spiritual needs, preferences, and concerns, both directly and symbolically [96]. Teams characterized by equilibrium and advancement serve as open systems. The boundaries in place are designed to be flexible and stable, accommodating the movement of families with seriously ill children based on their requirements. The team members are not susceptible to feeling overwhelmed by the family's grief, confusion, disorganization, despair, or suffering. They have the capacity to encapsulate these experiences. Their primary objective is to aid parents and children in acknowledging, articulating, and embracing their emotions while also facilitating their integration of various experiences and adjustment to a frequently challenging, uncertain, and unpredictable reality. Their role involves assisting families throughout the entire process of a child's illness, treatment, or passing and, in some instances, fostering enduring relationships during the lengthy period of mourning. Teams that encounter difficulties in areas such as boundary maintenance, goal setting, or time management are prone to establishing enmeshed or avoidant relationships with the patient and family [67]. The occurrence of an enmeshed relationship is a result of the team and family's inability to handle suffering, along with the potential or actual occurrence of death. They unite as a single entity and persist as undifferentiated, occasionally even after the child's recovery or demise. To provide an example, a team might seek families that deeply admire and celebrate it, whereas some families may rely on the team to preserve the memory of their departed child as a means of avoiding moving forward in life. Conversely, a relationship characterized by avoidance between a team and a family results in their partnership being reduced to a purely bureaucratic arrangement. It becomes a consumer-provider dynamic focused solely on handling practical matters, neglecting the emotional and spiritual dimensions of coping with a life-threatening illness. Relationships characterized by avoidance or enmeshment often indicate the team's and family's struggle to effectively cope with the difficulties associated with living with or dying from a life-threatening illness.

## 5.7 Teams Working Together

### 5.7.1 Principles, Practices, and Particular Challenges

It is customary for teams in pediatric palliative care to engage in collaboration with various professionals and teams. These encompass specialized teams that focus on disease-specific interventions, such as cystic fibrosis, oncology, and neuromuscular teams. Additionally, there are teams dedicated to organ transplantations and critical care interventions. Furthermore, there are teams involved in day-to-day care, such as home care, community care, hospice, and educational teams. In addition, palliative care teams establish a strong partnership with mental health and bereavement specialists who deliver counseling services to family members. The establishment of parallel collaborations with professionals, teams, organizations, and services is crucial in pediatric palliative care. Nonetheless, the successful implementation of such collaborations necessitates effective communication, meticulous planning, and the adoption of an approach known as "open teamwork," as discussed below [97]. While acknowledging the importance of other teams, all of these teams recognize their essential role in meeting the complex needs of children.

When dealing with life-threatening illnesses and their families, there may be instances where the specific issues they tackle and the responsibilities they undertake coincide. The allocation of care responsibilities may also change throughout the child's illness. As an illustration, the oncology team may encompass within their purview matters pertaining to pain management, symptom control, as well as the social and emotional well-being of the child and their family during curative treatment.

Nevertheless, as the disease advances and the potential for mortality arises, the oncology team may perceive the duty to manage pain and symptoms, as well as addressing the social and emotional requirements of the child and family, as more aligned with the palliative care team. The child and parents may not have any awareness or preference for this division and may wish for both teams to continue providing their services concurrently [96, 98].

Therefore, it is imperative that all teams participating in the care of these children and families demonstrate a shared commitment to an agreed-upon philosophy that also respects the families' choices. Frequently, families have a preference for an approach that combines disease-directed care with symptom-directed and supportive care [96, 99]. The constant presence of the potential for recurrence, worsening, and mortality is never far from the minds of children with life-threatening illnesses and their parents. Such thoughts frequently surface during instances where important decisions regarding further disease-oriented care and treatment are required. The difficulty is heightened not just by the inherent complexity of the decisions but also by the multitude of individuals who are both involved in and influenced by these decisions. It is the joint responsibility of teams to guide patients and families throughout the decision-making process. Just like families, all teams tasked with the care of children with life-threatening illnesses must grapple with the prospect of the children's demise. Although the primary focus of disease-oriented teams is combating mortality, it would be erroneous for them to disregard the likelihood of it occurring for a considerable portion of their patient population. In a similar vein, although palliative care teams recognize childhood mortality as inevitable in certain instances and acknowledge their constraints in reversing a terminal illness, they cannot disregard the fact that some team members, other collaborating teams, and the patients and families still perceive the battle against the disease. All individuals must refrain from making statements such as "Tomorrow may bring better circumstances" or "We are powerless to act" [67]. Although the prioritization of alleviating suffering persists, its complete eradication is unattainable. Throughout the diagnosis, relapses, and physical decline and notably in the terminal stage, the family endures an intense and frequently prolonged grieving process [100]. It is imperative for all teams working alongside these families to acknowledge that alleviating suffering requires more than quick fixes and predetermined interventions. It is imperative to provide support to patients and families in managing their losses and grief while also helping them develop the necessary resources and resilience to navigate the disease and cope with the child's passing.

## 5.8 The Team's Ability to Function with Competence

Every team faces multiple challenges in the face of uncertainty and grief that characterize the experiences of the children and families. Teams employ diverse strategies to address the anxiety and distress brought about by these realities. The presence of three fundamental conditions is highly correlated with the emergence of functional patterns. These commitments involve clearly defining goals and tasks for team members and providing a supportive environment for children, adolescents, families, and care providers. Additionally, they promote open teamwork through interdisciplinary collaborations [67].

### 5.8.1 Commitment

Care providers who perceive their services to seriously ill children and families as meaningful and valuable must demonstrate a high level of commitment when working in a field that causes increased distress. These professionals should acknowledge the potential and constraints of science in treating life-threatening illnesses and create circumstances that enhance the quality of life. Their dedication to this profession comprises two distinct elements: a dedication to a care philosophy characterized by specific, achievable, and well-defined objectives and responsibilities and a dedication to colleagues and the team. These goals and tasks are designed to foster the welfare and improve the quality of life for children, adolescents, families, and individuals of importance to them who hold significance in their lives. They contribute to the delineation of team members' obligations, duties, and tactics for achieving them, and if tasks are unclear or contradict one another, professionals are less likely to demonstrate commitment and are prone to assuming responsibilities that deviate from their intended tasks or role boundaries. One of the difficulties in the provision of care for children with life-threatening illnesses is the pursuit of ideal or unattainable standards of excellence. Realistic objectives recognize the constraints of care providers and teams. For example, sometimes death cannot be avoided nor life prolonged. In certain instances, despite the diligent efforts of everyone involved, the progression toward death can be characterized by suffering. Moreover, there are occasions when death transpires in traumatic conditions or when the family neglects to confront the impending reality of death. While it is of utmost importance for a team to strive toward guaranteeing a respectable quality of life for the entire family, as well as a dignified passing for the patient, the only commitment care providers can truly offer is the presence of a meaningful connection. In the context of that relationship, they will persist in being present, accessible, and capable of establishing continuity despite the presence of loss, separation, and suffering. To accomplish the intended objectives and foster a collaborative and supportive environment, it is crucial to display a strong commitment toward co-workers and the team. It is a common occurrence for professionals to face feelings of grief and distress while providing care to children with life-threatening illnesses. Recognizing the hardships faced by professionals and taking proactive measures involves team members openly discussing personal experiences and actively prioritizing their own well-being and that of their colleagues. When individuals are dedicated to their colleagues, they demonstrate care and concern through acts of solidarity and mutual assistance. Holding behaviors encompass acts that demonstrate care, kindness, and support.

Examples encompass actively listening to a colleague's personal encounters and challenges, providing constructive feedback rather than dispensing advice or therapy, and providing support to a co-worker during times of distress. These behaviors play a crucial role in fostering a culture of mutual support. Mutual support is marked by [67, 101]:

- The process of informational support involves the exchange of patient and family information, along with feedback on team operations, in order to enhance the quality of care and facilitate change or adaptation.
- The concept of practical support entails offering guidance, aid, or assistance to facilitate the accomplishment of specific tasks.
- The act of providing emotional support involves creating opportunities for team members to express their personal emotions and thoughts in a secure and nurturing environment, where they feel recognized, understood, and valued.
- Aid in the formation of meaning: the facilitation of opportunities for reflection and assimilation of work-related experiences to attribute significance and merge them into the team's narrative.

It is worth mentioning that while all forms of mutual support are imperative, the manner in which support is rendered should be tailored to the varying needs and preferences of care providers. The presence of mutual support has been identified as a determining factor in professionals' level of job satisfaction. According to studies, a key factor leading to professional burnout and turnover is not the team's exposure to multiple child deaths, no matter how distressing, but rather the team's lack of support for its members [67, 102]. Committed care providers demonstrate dedication to meaningful goals and tasks, depending on one another for the achievement of these goals while offering reciprocal support during the caregiving process.

### 5.8.2 Holding Environment

The concept of holding environment was initially introduced by Donald Winnicott, an English pediatrician and psychoanalyst. Winnicott emphasized the crucial role parents play in providing their infants with effective care, thereby influencing the child's psychosocial development [103]. Parents cultivate a nurturing atmosphere with well-defined boundaries that grants the infant a feeling of security from the outside world. Within this context, parents foster a sense of structure, consistency, and predictability, ultimately facilitating the child's transition from the secure parental bond to the gradually assimilated external world, to which the child adapts. Similarly, the team fosters within families a sense of safety, order, predictability, and continuity, all of which are crucial during times of crisis, ambiguity, uncertainty, and loss. Nevertheless, it is imperative for a team to establish a similar setting that ensures the well-being of its members. This can be achieved by fostering a secure organizational space where the stresses, conflicts, suffering, and hopes related to the difficulties of caring for children with life-threatening illnesses can be addressed. The significance of this cannot be overstated, as professionals' ability to effectively support children and families during a serious illness is greatly enhanced when they are supported by their team and organization [30]. Consistent exposure to mortality can exhaust a team's assets, leaving professionals to cope with their anguish and distress in solitude [67, 104]. With the establishment of a holding environment, care providers can experience a sense of safety amidst overwhelming experiences. They are able to acknowledge and accept their suffering as a natural part of their journey, seeking temporary support from understanding individuals who validate their emotions and have confidence in their capacity to navigate work-related difficulties. It is paradoxical that team members, when securely attached and supported by others, are able to develop self-reliance [105]. Intra-team relationships are defined by mature interdependence and are distinguished by a collective appreciation for autonomy and connectedness [104].

The presence of a holding environment does not lead to the disempowerment of care providers through excessive protection, nor does it provide an excuse for their inadequacies. On the contrary, it presents a sanctuary where individuals can seek refuge amidst distress, anxiety, anger, sadness, or fear. Furthermore, it serves as a stable anchor from which they can effectively process their experiences, proactively addressing difficulties and anxiety-inducing circumstances. The provision of a holding environment serves to fulfill five crucial functions for members of a team [67]:

The presence of a sense of safety establishes boundaries that safeguard team members against detrimental interferences from external factors such as organizational, bureaucratic, and financial limitations, as well as from internal sources including gossip or unwarranted blame. Within a secure setting, care providers have the liberty to openly communicate their feelings, thoughts, frustrations, and concerns, without the apprehension of being judged or criticized.

The ability to contain experiences refers to the empathetic understanding and acceptance of painful or threatening experiences, without dismissing, repressing, masking, distorting, or fragmenting them. In contrast to avoiding distressing feelings and experiences, the team actively embraces and openly confronts any anxiety, pain, or distress.

The process of elaborating experiences entails the exploration and assimilation of challenging experiences, losses, and frustrations. Its purpose is to prevent immobilization, particularly in circumstances characterized by trauma or heightened anxiety. The process involves disseminating information among team members who analyze the fundamental dynamics of a particular situation and utilize this information to grow both individually and collectively as a team. Elaboration enables individuals to adopt alternative perspectives in situations that induce anxiety, reframe distressing events, construct meaningful narratives, and enhance their understanding of themselves, others, and the team.

The regulation of distress and transformation of suffering offer team members the chance to manage their work, prioritize tasks, and reduce chaos, confusion, and distress. The aim is not to eradicate the inherent stressors in the care of children with life-threatening illnesses, but rather to effectively manage them and transform the inevitable suffering caused by loss and dying into meaningful outcomes. Through this approach, the team leverages its resources to cultivate resilience.

Promoting interconnectedness, interdependence, and a sense of belonging helps care providers avoid feelings of isolation and teaches them how to support others while receiving support themselves. The foundation of effective collaborations lies in mutual respect and shared responsibility, which encourage interdependence and empower autonomy.

The establishment of a holding environment inherently presents a potential risk for the team, as it may expose them to various forms of personal and collective suffering, such as fear, anxiety, despair, and powerlessness, induced by uncertainty, loss, and mortality, which are frequently regarded as excessively menacing. Despite the discomfort it may cause, confrontation is essential for processing and integrating experiences into the team's narrative, ultimately fostering progress. Nonetheless, there exist teams that are hesitant to assume this risk, impeding every deliberate endeavor to foster a nurturing environment by obstructing members from engaging in introspection and expressing unsettling emotions. Their actions contribute to the establishment of a culture that emphasizes invulnerability and omnipotence, thereby compromising the team's competence. Although a holding environment allows for the emergence of pain, it also acts as a countermeasure against the distress and affliction associated with the care of seriously ill children.

### 5.8.3 Interdisciplinary Collaboration and Open Teamwork

The team's competence is demonstrated by their ability to foster interdisciplinary collaboration among professionals with diverse expertise, rather than just coexisting or juxtaposing their services, but integrating them into a comprehensive care framework. Integration plays a central role in a relationship-centered approach, which aims to address the needs of a network of influential individuals who are both impacted by and impact the life of a seriously ill child.

Achieving the integration of services into a comprehensive framework relies on the cooperation of a unified team. The team fosters connections and collaborations with professionals, teams, organizations, or services in both the larger organization and the community. The team upholds boundaries that are both permeable and flexible, enabling the flow of information within and beyond its confines. The fostering of open teamwork is achieved through the establishment of a secure base by the team, from which its members can temporarily venture out to form coalitions with diverse groups and teams, ultimately integrating them into the team. By following this process, the team is able to holistically address the multifaceted physical, psychosocial, and spiritual needs of children and families that arise in various settings throughout the course of the illness. Effective collaboration is equally essential when the team is tasked with overseeing the transfer of patient care from pediatric specialists to adult specialists, which is a direct result of the increasing number of individuals diagnosed with life-threatening conditions during childhood who now survive into adulthood.

In general, collaborative teamwork encourages the implementation of initiatives and advancements while incorporating various approaches and services into a comprehensive care plan that benefits both the entire family and the individuals important to them. Open teamwork also allows care providers to gain perspective on how their services are perceived, aiding in the assessment of their impact on the community and the societal benefits derived from their contribution.

### 5.8.4 Assessing the Team's Ability to Function with Competence

Teams represent complex systems that undergo constant transformation and development. By recognizing that their competence is improved by favorable working conditions that foster commitment, a conducive environment, and collaborative teamwork, professionals can assess the extent to which these conditions are developed and identify areas that need attention and further improvement. In an ideal scenario, the establishment of these three conditions gives rise to an equilateral triangle, wherein the base symbolizes a commitment to a care-based philosophy, clearly defined objectives and tasks, and mutual camaraderie. In their study, Ketchum and Trist emphasize the centrality of work commitment in people's lives [106]. The stronger the commitment, the greater the likelihood that team members will trust one another in establishing a holding environment. This environment can effectively contain their experiences and emotions, fostering a willingness to take risks and engage in collaborative efforts with other professionals and teams, ultimately benefiting their patients. Similarly, when a holding environment effectively ensures team members' safety, order, predictability, and continuity during challenging periods, their commitment to shared objectives and colleagues intensifies. In the same vein, the willingness of care providers to engage in interdisciplinary collaborations, both within and outside of their team, directly correlates with their personal and professional enrichment. This, in turn, reinforces their dedication to their job and team. It is evident that the described conditions are closely linked, and advancements in one area contribute to advancements in the others.

The ensuing data illustrates the obstacles faced by two teams in their efforts to create work environments that promote competence. Within a single pediatric palliative care team, professionals demonstrate dedication to clearly defined objectives and responsibilities while benefiting from a supportive environment that fosters a sense of security, enabling them to openly discuss cases and express their emotional reactions, concerns, or errors. In lieu of bearing hardship in solitude, team members rely on the knowledge and feedback of their peers. Nonetheless, in the team as portrayed herein, a disparity emerges between the imperative for cultivating and mutual bolstering and the present holding environment, which, although extant, is yet to attain full maturation. Hence, team members demonstrate a reluctance to engage in substantial risk-taking as they lack confidence in their team's ability to provide assistance during times of intense distress or crisis. The team's preference for a shorter line of open teamwork suggests their reluctance to engage in collaborations with other professionals in the larger organization and community. This has implications for families, who are unable to access essential services, and for care providers, who are solely reliant on their own resources, leading to both groups being confined to an insular environment. Although this environment offers a certain degree of security and safeguard, it simultaneously marginalizes the remainder of the societal populace. In the absence of regular evaluation, enhancement, or alteration of team goals, tasks, and practices, their strong commitment remains rigid. Additionally, the extent of one's devotion to colleagues and co-workers is subject to change depending on the nature of collaborations that arise within or outside the team, at any given moment.

## 5.9 Directions for Research, Education, and Practice

There is a lack of professionals capable of addressing the diverse needs of children and families facing life-threatening illnesses. Providing care for children with life-threatening illnesses necessitates a comprehensive and diverse set of tools and knowledge, coupled with a profound and enduring understanding of the challenges and achievements experienced by both the children and their families. The mere act of assembling a team of exceptionally qualified and extensively trained professionals does not suffice in meeting the needs of both children and families. The development and maintenance of team competency are essential in providing quality care for these children and families. The attainment and maintenance of team competence necessitates not only focusing on the team's care for the children and families but also on its care for itself and its members. A notable scarcity of literature exists regarding the provision of care by teams to patients, families, and their own members. With the aim of filling this gap, our suggestion for a research agenda involves the comprehensive study of care providers' and teams' experiences. In a more specific manner, we must take into consideration the following.

This analysis examines the development of teams, focusing on the professional, interpersonal, and institutional challenges and opportunities that arise in teamwork. It also considers the requisite skills and abilities needed to achieve and sustain team competency.

What is the nature of different service delivery models (such as palliative care teams, hospice teams, disease-directed teams, integrated palliative care teams, and disease-directed teams), and what are their associated costs? Such studies have the potential to form a basis for evidence-based recommendations regarding care delivery in different community settings. The examination places emphasis on the nature of relationships that develop among individuals, comprising of care providers, patients, and family members. Moreover, it acknowledges the importance of the relationships between teams and families, highlighting the significance of trust, decision-making processes, smooth transitions, and the uninterrupted delivery of care. These factors are recognized as important results of relationships between professionals, patients, and parents.

The influence of professionals and their teams on the care they deliver and the reciprocal impact they encounter are very important. These studies should encompass both the positive outcomes of caregiving, such as personal development and the acquisition of leadership abilities, and the negative consequences of their experiences, which may involve anxiety, burnout, or compassion fatigue.

How does the culture and society in which these teams operate influence their capacity to develop and meet the needs of patients and families? Furthermore, there is a demand for increased training in the successful execution of team practices. Despite the rise in available training opportunities and programs in palliative care, there remains a significant lack of offerings focused on team dynamics, functioning, and growth in the context of serious illness and death. We highly recommend program organizers to capitalize on the diverse presence of individuals from various professional backgrounds, skills, and experiences by incorporating sessions that tackle teamwork-related issues. Additionally, we recommend the creation of educational resources and initiatives that showcase and promote collaboration among practitioners from different scientific and professional fields. It is essential to give priority to the development of materials and programs that offer techniques for:

- Engaging in the elicitation and discussion of responses to challenging situations and relationships.
- Deliberation of challenging matters, encompassing both clinical and managerial aspects.
- Encouraging teams to engage in self-monitoring and reflection while delivering services.

Valuable resources for the development of materials and programs include the Children's Project on Palliative/Hospice Services (the ChiPPS Project), which is sponsored by the National Hospice and Palliative Care Association [107, 108]. Evaluation of educational and training programs, similar to the teams themselves, is necessary. Efforts are underway to develop tools for evaluating palliative care curricula; however, further work is necessary to encompass diverse disciplines and program formats [108]. It is advisable to offer training on assessing the team's contribution to service delivery, which teams can utilize in their interactions. These approaches can also be utilized to assess the immediate and long-term impacts of new or existing team strategies, such as support groups, debriefing sessions, and retreats. Additionally, they could offer a substantiated foundation for the sustainability or cessation of said practices. Various researchers and clinicians have highlighted the importance of conducting research on interventions aimed at preventing compassion fatigue and burnout [108].

# Managing Symptoms in Pediatric Palliative Care

# 6

**Guidelines for Symptom Control**

The guidelines of managing symptoms encompass the following:

1. In-Depth Evaluation and Treatment of the Root Cause: Whenever feasible, it is essential to thoroughly assess and treat the underlying cause of the symptoms.
2. Consideration of Non-pharmacological Management Techniques: Depending on the symptom, non-pharmacological management techniques should be considered. These may include dietary modifications, adjustments in positioning, and the use of diversion techniques such as art or music.
3. Pharmacological Management for Symptom Relief: In certain cases, pharmacological interventions directed at symptom relief are necessary. For instance, anti-emetic medications may be prescribed to alleviate nausea and vomiting.
4. Effective Communication and Reassurance: It is crucial to provide clear and thorough explanations to both the child and their family, along with reassurance throughout.
5. Multidisciplinary Team Role: In order to provide effective palliative care, it is essential to involve a multidisciplinary team. This acknowledges that the needs of both the child and their family cannot be adequately addressed by a single discipline. To adequately meet the diverse palliative care needs of the child and their family, it is imperative to involve disciplines such as a physician, an advanced practice nurse or clinical nurse specialist, a pediatrician, and a social worker [62, 110].

## 6.1 Addressing Pain Management in Children

### 6.1.1 Introduction

Assessing pain is a complex task, particularly when factoring in the distinct growth and developmental stages encountered in the management of various age groups. Evaluating pain in infants and children presents additional challenges, which have precipitated the development of numerous tools and scoring systems tailored to specific age brackets. It is paramount to acknowledge that children proceeding toward the end of life may experience symptoms beyond pain. These can encompass fatigue, diminished energy, breathlessness, loss of appetite, nausea, vomiting, sleep disturbances, anxiety, and additional symptoms. The interrelation of these symptoms often exacerbates their impact on the individual's well-being [109, 111].


N. Javadi-Pashaki et al., *Interdisciplinary Pediatric Palliative Care*,
https://doi.org/10.1007/978-981-97-9587-1_6

### 6.1.2 Pain

Pain as the fifth vital sign should be considered and checked routinely. The International Association for the Study of Pain defined pain as "an unpleasant sensory and emotional experience associated with actual or potential tissue damage, or described in terms of such damage" [112].

#### 6.1.2.1 Pain Theories

The specificity theory of pain, initially proposed by René Descartes during the sixteenth century, stands as one of the original theories on pain. According to the statement, there is a direct correlation between the intensity of pain and the extent of tissue injury. The unidimensional approach to pain suggests that analgesics can effectively treat all forms of pain. Dr. Henry Beecher acknowledged the limitations of this theory amidst the Second World War, observing that merely one-third of soldiers admitted to a combat hospital exhibited significant pain that warranted the administration of morphine. He made a remark about the occurrence of a discrepancy between the intensity of pain and the severity of the injury in specific circumstances. In 1965, Melzack and Wall put forth the gate control theory of pain, which posited the existence of a spinal cord mechanism that governs the transmission of pain signals from the periphery to the brain. The theory redirected focus from the peripheral source of injury to the spinal cord and brain. This study offered the initial physiological explanation for how psychological interventions, like distraction or relaxation, can effectively alleviate pain. Subsequent to their research, a progressively multidimensional perspective on pain was embraced, and healthcare professionals currently acknowledge that pain perception is influenced by various factors (the neuromatrix theory of pain).

Dame Cicely Saunders was aware that there are other crucial factors that can influence the perception of pain. In parallel with the work of others, she developed the concept of "total pain" from her understanding that the origins of pain may be:

- Physical.
- Social.
- Psychological.
- Spiritual [113, 114] (Fig. 6.1).

The notion of total pain has emerged as a fundamental principle in the field of palliative care. It acknowledges the fact that cancer-related pain is frequently a multifaceted and persistent form of pain, stemming from various concurrent factors. The successful management of cancer pain necessitates a comprehensive approach that encompasses the patient's emotional well-being and physical pain treatment. Therefore, the delivery of analgesics should be accompanied by the provision of emotional, social, and spiritual support [11].

#### 6.1.2.2 Physical Pain in Patients with Cancer

Pain is a prevalent and dreaded symptom associated with cancer. Numerous individuals diagnosed with non-malignant, life-threatening conditions also experience significant pain. Despite the existence of effective pain control methods, a considerable number of individuals still experience insufficient pain relief. Pain associated with cancer can be classified as either acute or chronic, with additional distinctions for chronic pain [30].

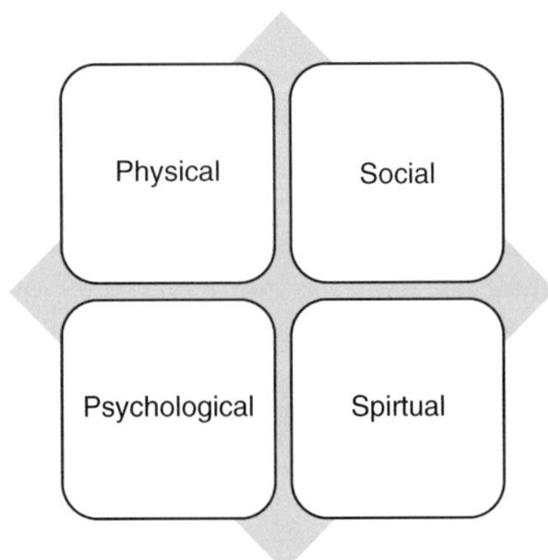


**Fig. 6.1** Concept of Total Pain. This figure is researcher-made design and has not been adapted from any resource

#### 6.1.2.3 Breakthrough Pain

Transiently, there is a surge in pain intensity known as breakthrough pain, surpassing the pre-existing background pain. Typically, breakthrough pain is associated with underlying pain. There are three distinct categories of breakthrough pain that have been outlined:

- Incident pain refers to pain that is associated with any type of movement, whether it is voluntary or involuntary.
- Idiopathic or spontaneous pain occurs without any identifiable cause.
- Failure observed at the termination of the dosage, just prior to the scheduled analgesia administration. Frequently underestimated as genuine breakthrough pain.

Breakthrough pain is prevalent in more than 50% of patients diagnosed with cancer, and it also manifests in patients with non-malignant conditions. This represents a negative prognostic factor, with potential consequences including diminished functioning, increased anxiety and depression, and extended hospitalization periods. In order to achieve optimal pain control, it is essential that all patients receiving opioids have access to breakthrough analgesia [115].

#### 6.1.2.4 Assessment of Pain

Examining pain in infants and children is done through three types of behavioral, physiological, and self-report measures, and its performance depends on the child's cognitive and speech ability.

- Physiological indicators should be used to assess pain in infants and also in children who have an endotracheal tube or who are neurologically damaged.
- Physiological indicators include increase in heart rate, increase in breathing rate, decrease in arterial blood oxygen saturation, increase in blood sugar, and pupil dilation and change in body color (change in skin mosaic color, pallor).
- Behavioral indicators of pain includes, frowning, poor feeding, insomnia, stiffening of the limbs, and movements of the limbs in infants; verbal or physical anger toward the painful place in toddlers; the ability to express pain but magical thinking gets in the way in preschoolers; and can express pain but are influenced by cultural beliefs in school age.
- Self-reporting indicators: Children over 3 years old have the ability to self-report pain [116].

#### 6.1.2.5 Pain Measurement Tools in Children

Tools used for measurement of pain in children and infants based on behavioral scales (such as facial expression, body position, facial expression or crying), physiological (such as heart rate or breathing or arterial blood oxygen saturation), and self-reporting (pain expression by child). Children less than 4 years old do not have the ability to self-report pain (they are not able to determine the level of their pain, and the nurse or his caregiver must determine the level of pain from the facial expression or physiological indicators) [116].

**Numeric rating scale (NRS):** This scale for pain is more common than others. The person rates their pain using a 0–10 or 0–5 scale. Zero means no pain, and 5 or 10 means the worst pain condition. These pain intensity levels may be assessed after initial treatment or periodically after treatment. It is used for children over 5 years old and adults, and the maximum score is 10 [117].

**Wong-Baker faces scale:** It is used for children over 3 years old. The maximum score is 10 [116].

**FLACC scale:** It is one of the most common tools for measuring pain. It is used for infants from 2 months to children of 7 years, as well as children who are unable to express their pain verbally. In this tool, five areas of facial expression, leg posture, activity, crying, and ability to calm the child/infant are checked, and the maximum score is 10 [116] (Table 6.1).

**Table 6.1** FLACC scale

| | Scoring | | |
|---|---|---|---|
| Category | 0 | 1 | 2 |
| Face | No particular expression or smile | Occasional grimace or frown, withdrawn disinterested | Frequent to constant quivering chin, clenched jaw |
| Leg | Normal position or relaxed | Uneasy, restless, tense | Kicking or legs drawn up |
| Activity | Lying quietly, normal position moves easily | Squirming, shifting back and forth, tense | Arched, rigid, or jerking |
| Cry | No cry | Moans or whimpers | Crying steadily, screams, sobs, frequent complaints |
| Consolability | Content, relaxed | Reassured by occasional touching, hugging or being talked to, distractable | Difficult to console or comfort |

**Table 6.2** CRIES scale

| | 0 | 1 | 2 |
|---|---|---|---|
| Crying | None | High-pitched | Inconsolable |
| Required $O_2$ | None | <30% $FiO_2$ needed | >30% $FiO_2$ needed |
| Increased vital signs | Normal HR and BP | Increased HR and BP <20% | Increased HR and BP >20% |
| Expression | Normal | Grimace | Grimace and grunt |
| Sleeplessness | None | Wakes frequently | Awake constantly |

**Table 6.3** CHEOPS scale

| Score | 0 | 1 | 2 |
|---|---|---|---|
| Cry | No cry | Moaning, crying | Scream |
| Facial | Smiling | Composed | Grimace |
| Verbal | Positive | None or other complaints | Pain complaints |
| Torso | Neutral | Shifting, tense, upright | Restrained |
| Legs | Neutral | Kicks, squirm, drawn up | Restrained |
| Touch | Not touching | Reach, touch, grab | Restrained |

**CRIES scale:** It is used for babies over 32 weeks and after surgery. It examines five domains including crying, oxygen demand, changes in vital signs, facial expression, and restlessness. The maximum score is 10. Painkillers are recommended for a pain score of 6 and above [118] (Table 6.2).

**CHEOPS scale:** It is used for children under 3 years of age or children who are unable to express pain verbally. This tool is also used to measure postoperative pain. This instrument examines six behaviors, including crying, speech, body posture, touch, and feet. Score 4 indicates the absence of pain, and score 13 indicates severe pain [119] (Table 6.3).

**PIPP scale:** It is used for premature babies and measures criteria including fetal age, ability to close eyes, manner of behavior, nasolabial fold, heart rate, oxygen saturation, and eyebrow protrusion. A score of 0 indicates no pain, and a score of 21 indicates severe pain [120].

**Oucher scale.** This tool is one of the most reliable, oldest, and most widely used self-report scales of children's pain intensity and was developed by Bayer to evaluate the pain intensity of children aged 3–12 years.

This tool contains six pictures of a child's face with different intensities of pain, which are placed vertically and based on the least to the most severe pain from the bottom to the top and are graded from 1 to 6 (1 is no pain, and 6 is the most severe pain) [116].

#### 6.1.2.6 Pain Management

The primary aim of pain management is to improve the quality of life for both the child and their family by relieving pain. This is achieved through a combination of pharmacological and non-pharmacological approaches. This entails a thorough assessment and the development of a customized care plan to meet the specific needs of the child.

#### 6.1.2.7 The Fundamental Principles of Pain Management

1. Undergo a comprehensive assessment and tackle the underlying issue when possible, considering the physical, psychological, social, and spiritual aspects.
2. Implement non-pharmacological strategies for managing pain, which may include methods such as massage, thermal therapy, and participation in activities such as play, art, or music.
3. Selecting the appropriate analgesic and determining the optimal dosage are critical components.
4. Consistent administration of analgesics is essential for both pain prevention and treatment.
5. Provide comprehensive written guidelines to the family regarding the dosage and frequency of administration.
6. Periodically evaluate the levels of pain experienced by the individual and meticulously review the approach to pain management.
7. Consider and address other factors that may potentially increase the intensity of pain, including anxiety or fear.

#### 6.1.2.8 Pharmacological Management of Pain in Pediatric

Nonsteroidal anti-inflammatory drugs (NSAIDs) serve as the primary cornerstone in the management of pain. However, it is important to acknowledge that the utilization of non-pharmacological interventions can also be beneficial for certain children. Nevertheless, in the majority of cases, the administration of pain medications is deemed essential. The fundamental principle underpinning the pharmacological management of pain is tailored according to the individual's pain threshold, and dosage is adjusted based on the specific condition. This approach involves a sequential series of evaluations to fine-tune the selection and administration of medications, aiming to strike an optimal balance between pain alleviation and potential adverse effects. The World Health Organization (WHO) has introduced a valuable framework for drug selection in the treatment of both acute and chronic pain, referred to as the "analgesic ladder" [121, 122].

1. **Choosing appropriate route**

For the administration of analgesia, the oral route is generally considered to be the most efficacious method. However, alternative routes must be considered in the cases of pediatric patients who are comatose, who are unable to swallow, or who experience recurrent episodes of vomiting. Other available routes encompass buccal, intranasal, rectal, subcutaneous (SC), intramuscular (IM) (which should be strictly avoided), and intravenous (IV) route, topical application (directly applied to the skin), and spinal or epidural nerve block.

2. **Around the clock**

It is imperative to administer analgesics at predetermined intervals or at fixed durations if the child experiences persistent pain. This approach is more effective than the as-needed principle (PRN), wherein treatment is contingent upon the onset of pain in the child. Adopting the "as needed" approach can exacerbate pain and anxiety, stemming from the apprehension of not being able to mitigate the pain effectively. The timing between doses is customized based on the duration of the drug's action; for instance, oral opioids may require a 4-h interval for effective relief. Adherence to a regular dosing schedule offers superior pain management compared to addressing each new episode of pain independently. Furthermore, a consistent dosing regimen at reduced doses is more efficient in pain control than resorting to larger doses for each subsequent episode of pain.

3. **Individualized dose to each child**

The administration of pain management should be personalized for each child, with the understanding that a standardized dosage regimen will not be effective across all children. Adjustments should be made to medication and dosage based on the child's response and potential adverse effects.

4. **Using the WHO ladder**

Principal guidelines encompass the utilization of the World Health Organization's distinct three-level pain scale (mild, moderate, severe) in the management of chronic pain, which proves particularly beneficial for pediatric patients. This methodology involves the selection of analgesics to be administered based on the child's pain intensity level [123] (Fig. 6.2).

- For mild to moderate pain levels (1–3 on a scale), it is advisable to initially recommend non-opioid analgesics, such as paracetamol or nonsteroidal anti-inflammatory drugs (NSAIDs) like ibuprofen.
- When managing moderate to severe pain (4–7 on the scale), it may be appropriate to consider a low-dose morphine regimen, which is 50% of the typical initial dosage. This can be utilized in higher tiers of the analgesic ladder, either alone or in conjunction with other analgesic strategies. It is important to note that the use of opioids like codeine and tramadol in pediatric patients should be avoided, as there is a scarcity of evidence supporting their efficacy and safety in this population.
- In cases of severe pain (8–10 on the scale), opioids should be the primary choice for the management of acute severe pain, with morphine often being the drug of choice. This regimen can also be adopted in higher tiers of the analgesic ladder, either independently or with the inclusion of other analgesic interventions.

The prescription of specific analgesic strategies should always be tailored to the severity of the pain and may need to be adjusted as pain severity fluctuates. Additionally, always avoid combined use of weak opioid with strong opioids when they compete with each other (Table 6.4).

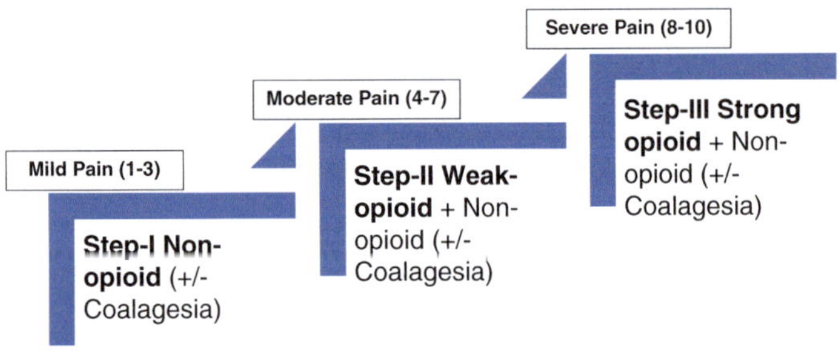


**Fig. 6.2** World Health Organization pain ladder. This figure is researcher-made design and has not been adapted from any resource

**Table 6.4** Common opioids and non-opioid to treat pain in children

| Pain severity | Type of opioid | Drug name | Dose |
|---|---|---|---|
| 1–3 | Non-opioid | Paracetamol | 10–15 mg/kg in 4–6 h |
| 4–7 | Weak opioid | Low-dose morphine<br>Tramadol (>12 years) | 0.05–0.1 mg/kg in every 4 h<br>1–2 mg/kg in every 6 h |
| 8–10 | Strong opioid | Morphine | Oral: 0.1–0.2 mg/kg in every 4 h<br>IV bolus: 0.1 mg/kg<br>IV infusion: 20 μg/kg/h |

### 6.1.3 Co-Analgesics or Adjuvants

Co-analgesics or adjuvants are drugs that have analgesic properties and can be used in combination with any analgesic included in the WHO pain ladder, although their primary purpose is not pain relief. Co-analgesics are particularly useful in dealing with neuropathic pain. Some commonally used adjuvants includes corticosteroids, anticonvulsants, beta-blocker, antispasmodics, and muscle relaxants, e.g., diazepam, baclofen, etc. [124].

#### 6.1.3.1 Morphine Use in Pediatric

- Administering morphine to children begins with an initial dose of morphine sulfate syrup orally to alleviate pain.
- The oral administration of morphine necessitates dosing every 4 h, as its effects are transient. In infants and patients suffering from hepatic or renal impairment, the interval between doses can extend to 6–8 h. The standard starting oral dosage of morphine sulfate is 0.2 mg/kg every 4 h. It is imperative to maintain a consistent administration schedule rather than dispensing morphine on an "as needed" basis.
- Additional doses, referred to as breakthrough doses (BTDs), may be administered when a child experiences pain preceding the scheduled regular dosage. The breakthrough dose is typically equivalent to 50–100% of the standard dose. Given that morphine's onset of action can take up to 30 min, it is advisable to avoid administering the maximum dose within this timeframe of the scheduled dose.
- Morphine is considered an effective analgesic due to its lack of a "ceiling effect." Consequently, should the current dosage not sufficiently manage pain, the dosage can be escalated. There exists no maximum oral dosage of morphine in the context of chronic pain management, and it is appropriate to incrementally increase the dosage to enhance pain relief. In instances where morphine must be discontinued after a period exceeding 10–14 days, a gradual reduction in dosage is essential to mitigate withdrawal symptoms.
- Morphine is widely regarded as an appropriate medication for the management of moderate to severe pain in children undergoing palliative care [125].

#### 6.1.3.2 Morphine Side Effect Management in Pediatric

The common side effects in child using morphine are as follows:

- Short-duration reactions, including drowsiness and sedation, tend to subside within the range of 48–72 h. Sometime child can develop nausea and vomiting, which can last for less than a week and managed by starting antiemetic (ondansetron for older children and metoclopramide (Maxolon) in infants) before using morphine.
- Ongoing side effects include constipation, managed with laxative lactulose or sorbitol use as a prophylactic dose.
- Some of the rare side effects include hypersensitivity, pruritus (itchy skin), and urinary retention also managed with medication [126].

#### 6.1.3.3 Challenges in Providing Appropriate Pain Management in Pediatric Palliative Care

- Ignoring the pain, including refusing to acknowledge its existence.
- Ignoring the widespread nature of pain, including its psychological, social, and cultural dimensions.
- Concerns about causing harm and experiencing adverse effects.
- Concerns about developing addiction and misuse.
- Concerns about the pain being misused.
- Exclusion of other non-drug treatments.
- Parents denying the pain, falsely believing it is a sign of worsening condition.
- Patients and parents believing that the pain is intractable and therefore not treated by the healthcare team [127, 128].

#### 6.1.3.4 Non-pharmacological Methods of Pain Relief

**Distraction Techniques**

Distraction entails involving the child in a diverse range of activities aimed at diverting their attention from the pain and anxiety that accompanies it. Illustrations of deviant activities comprise the following:

- Engage in activities such as listening to music, singing, playing games, watching TV or videos, or concentrating on an image while counting.
- Select appropriate activities that align with the child's developmental needs. While children in severe pain may not be easily diverted, it would be erroneous to conclude that their pain has ceased if they display signs of distraction.
- Play music for the child, play cartoons, or let them play games with the mobile phone.
- Tell the child to take deep breaths and exhale until you say "stop."
- Tell the child to make bubbles with the bubble machine and make the bubbles go away from him as an example.
- Ask the child to yawn or say "ouch" and teach him to say it as loudly or softly as it hurts.
- Tell jokes or cartoons for the child, tell funny stories, or use toys that make the child laugh.
- Allow the child to read books and play with his friends.
- Use binoculars and ask the child to focus and ask him: "Does he see something different each time?" [129].

**Relaxation Techniques**

If the child is younger:

- Hold the baby in a comfortable position.
- Then rock the baby in your arms like a cradle (back and forth).
- Repeat one or two words slowly, for example, "Mommy is here."

If the child is older:

- Ask the child to take a deep breath and exhale slowly and let the air slowly leave his mouth. Then ask him to yawn.
- Help the child get into a comfortable position. For example, put a pillow under his neck or knees.
- Do relaxation on the body parts for him. First, start with the toes and teach the child to relax and let go of that part, and also ask him to tell us the next part by himself, for example, "Now go to the leg part" or "Go to the right-hand part," and ask him first. Contract that part and then relax.
- During relaxation, tell the child to keep his eyes open because it helps the child to follow your instructions better [130].

**Guided Imaginary**

Tell the child:

Today I want to do an exercise together:

- First, think of a scene or scene you like.
- Ask him to describe that scene. For example, do you see beautiful colors? Is there a cool breeze? Do you listen to soothing music?
- Ask the child to write them down or record his voice.
- Encourage the child to focus on just one favorite scene (and recall it, by looking at his handwriting or audio recording) when he is in pain.
- Combine this exercise with deep breathing or music.

Thinking positive:

- Teach the child to repeat positive statements to himself when in pain such as "I will feel better," "I will go home," and "I will feel better and I can eat ice cream or pizza."

Stop thinking:

- Teach the child to think about the positive aspects of the painful procedure, for example, "Finally this work will be finished."
- Reassure the child that "if I think about something else, it won't hurt too much."
- Teach the child to repeat short and positive sentences with you, for example, "good vein, little pain, short procedure, good nurse, going home, seeing father, brother and sister."

- Teach the child to repeat these short sentences whenever he feels pain [131].

**Behavioral Contract**

**Informal:** For 4- or 5-year-old children that includes:

- Using tokens, stars, or cartoon stickers as prizes.
- If a child does not cooperate and is aggressive, set a limited time with a timer that the child can see and say that you must do this procedure during this time.
- Encourage the child's cooperation with a reward if the procedure is completed within the allotted time.

**Formal:** A formal written contract for older children that includes:

- Identify rewards or consequences that are reinforcing.
- Specify the objectives to be evaluated.
- Determine the commitment requirements for both parties (e.g., use a timer during the procedure, and when you turn it on, the nurse has no right to be rude and the stubborn child must be patient until the procedure is finished) [132].

**Skin Stimulation**

Skin stimulation includes gently massaging the painful area and surrounding skin and holding or rocking the child. Touch acts as a stimulus and causes it to compete with pain stimuli transmitted from peripheral nerves to the spinal cord. These measures may reduce the child's pain. Swaddles and blankets may calm an anxious baby by reducing tactile stimulation and movement behaviors [30, 133].

**Other Techniques**

- Infants engage in activities such as embracing, stroking, using pacifiers, and receiving massages.
- The activities for toddlers include massage, storytelling, bubbles, tactile experiences, holding and swinging, and listening to music.
- Elementary students actively participate in games, stories, music, imaginative play, hero role-playing, and watching TV or videos. They can benefit from practices such as regular breathing, muscle relaxation, guided imagery, discussing pleasurable experiences, engaging in games, listening to the radio, or watching TV or videos.
- Adolescents can utilize various strategies including regular breathing, muscle relaxation, guided imagery, social interactions with visitors, participation in games, TV viewing, and listening to the radio or CD player [132].

### 6.1.4 Summary

Pain in children is frequently underestimated and inadequately managed. The proper management of pain can greatly improve the quality of life for children who have incurable illnesses. The implementation of enhanced education and training programs for healthcare providers may result in a positive influence on pain management in children. A diverse team of specialists who possess qualities such as open-mindedness, attentiveness, accessibility, adaptability, innovation, resourcefulness, and compassion can help in reducing discomfort for the child and their family. Open and interactive discussions regarding treatment goals, available alternatives, and their corresponding adverse effects can assist patients and their families in choosing the most suitable approach that aligns with their preferences. By maintaining the patient and their family's dignity and ensuring they are not alone in their struggles, we can alleviate their collective suffering.

## 6.2 Managing Gastrointestinal-Associated Symptoms

### 6.2.1 Introduction

Additionally, non-oncology pediatric patients displaying gastrointestinal symptoms no less severe than those observed in oncology pediatric patients were included in the examination. Vomiting and constipation are significant components of home care for children and adolescents with life-limiting illnesses, specifically in relation to gastrointestinal symptoms. It is crucial to determine various causes and obtain prompt relief from symptoms. Due to gastrointestinal symptoms, numerous pediatric patients endure significant suffering at the end of their lives. The most common symptoms among children with incurable disease such as cancer are cachexia and anorexia (71–100%), constipation (39–50%), nausea and vomiting (50–57%), and diarrhea (21–40%) [134, 135].

## 6.2.2 Nausea and Vomiting

The manifestation of these symptoms may influence other pivotal decisions related to care, in conjunction with the distress experienced by nausea and vomiting toward the terminal phase of life. Should nausea and vomiting prove to be unyielding or inadequately addressed within the outpatient setting, for example, patients may choose to transition to inpatient care rather than remaining under home care. Furthermore, nausea and vomiting can exert a considerable physical functioning on the capacity of children to embrace the remainder of their lives and attend to their spiritual and existential requirements, similar to the impact of other symptoms at the end of life [136].

### 6.2.2.1 Assessment

Like any other symptoms, the presence of nausea and vomiting necessitates evaluation. Evaluate the intensity, occurrence, initiation, and length of nausea, along with any accompanying vomiting. Assess the vomiting pattern, content, and volume with care and also evaluate both provocation and palliative factors. Past medical/treatment history including chemotherapy, radiation, current medication, and constipation will help to determine what might be causing nausea. Blood analyses, including liver function tests and renal function tests, as well as electrolyte levels, serum calcium, and additional parameters, are conducted to identify the underlying cause.

### 6.2.2.2 Management

Assess for dehydration, reassure, calm the environment, avoid the smell of food, and feed the child frequently in small quantities that are appealing to the child are non-pharmacological measures.

Serotonin antagonists (diphenhydramine + metoclopramide) are one type of pharmacological intervention useful in symptom relief. Ondansetron can be injected or taken orally for nausea and vomiting caused by chemotherapy-induced nausea and vomiting. Recommendation to use protan pump inhibitors and antacids in condition such as gastritis. Sometime anxiolytic drugs are used for anticipatory nausea and anxiety.

## 6.2.3 Constipation

Constipation frequently serves as a significant source of discomfort and suffering among children facing death. The evaluation and management of constipation, along with the related unease, can further intensify sentiments of diminished dignity, especially in the older adolescent and young adult population. A main objective ought to be prevention. Determine the potential causes of constipation, inactivity, reduced mobility, and the use of medications like opiates, anticholinergics, iron, and so on. Limited oral intake and complications of the underlying disease such as fecal withholding due to anorectal issues also lead to constipation [137].

### 6.2.3.1 Assessment

- The recurrence rate of evacuations, the regularity of bowel movements, and the associated pain during defecation should all be meticulously documented in a detailed medical history.
- Symptoms such as abdominal discomfort, nausea, emesis, and a diminished appetite are indicative of constipation and warrant a thorough evaluation.
- In the course of an abdominal examination, rigid stools may be felt. For children who are unable to communicate effectively verbally,

the process of abdominal palpation may induce discomfort or lead to facial expressions of distress.

- While it is often possible to diagnose and manage constipation effectively without conducting a digital examination, a rectal examination is a valuable tool for assessing rectal tone and identifying the presence of feces in the rectum.

#### 6.2.3.2 Management

Pharmacological interventions encompass a range of therapies aimed at addressing constipation, including the administration of stool softeners such as docusate. Additionally, the use of osmotic agents, such as lactulose or magnesium sulfate, is employed. Stimulants, including senna and bisacodyl, are also utilized in the management of constipation. Suppositories and enemas are examples of rectal medications that, like oral medications, soften stools or encourage their evacuation. Non-pharmacological interventions includes fiber rich diet, increase fluid consumption and encourage for the mobility [138].

### 6.2.4 Diarrhea

Diarrhea is a debilitating and embarrassing condition that is characterized by an abnormal looseness of the stools (increased liquidity or decreased consistency). Children who have diarrhea that is uncontrolled are more likely to become dehydrated, have an imbalance of electrolytes, have skin breakdown, and feel tired.

#### 6.2.4.1 Management

Identifying treatable causes of diarrhea, such as enteral or non-enteral infection, malabsorption, and medication-induced diarrhea (antibiotics, excessive laxative use, chemotherapy), is the first step in treatment.

#### 6.2.4.2 Management of Diarrhea

In-case of diarrhea, maintaining the hydration level with using Oral Rehydration Solution (ORS) and correction of electrolyte and acid-base imbalances with IV fluids (if severe). If the cause of infection is bacterial or parasitic, antibiotics are recommended. In acute diarrhea, anti-diarrheal medications should be avoided. Antispasmodic medications are the best option for managing colicky pain. Take the laxative under physician supervision. Educate and demonstrate proper handwashing techniques, and encourage parents to avoid contaminated food [139].

### 6.2.5 Anorexia and Cachexia

Losing weight and not getting enough nutrition are often seen as unavoidable consequences in children as they grow older, and they can sometimes lead to worse health outcomes, increased sadness, and higher mortality. Not being able to eat (anorexia) or losing weight without wanting to (cachexia) can affect how well a child lives and can also worsen the symptoms that come with not getting enough nutrients. Food and eating can be very important to the child and their families. Children need more energy and nutrients than adults because they are in the phase of growth, development and maturity [140, 141].

#### 6.2.5.1 Management

When implementing a therapeutic approach for cachexia, it is equally crucial to evaluate and address the concurrent illness and psychological distress that commonly coexist. The treatment plan should encompass the goals of both the child and their family, with a focus on maximizing quality of life and an assessment of the current disease stage. Unfortunately, the optimal approach to treating cachexia is through the cure of cancer or end-stage disease. In case of any obstruction, parenteral nutrition and without obstruction tube feedings might give solace to children and the families. The majority of weight gain is attributed to an increase in adipose tissue, and supplemental hypercaloric nutrition administered via an IV or feeding tube has little effect on increasing skeletal muscle mass [142, 143].

### 6.2.6 Summary

Children frequently experience end-of-life gastrointestinal symptoms. The process of diagnosing and treating common symptoms encompasses both pharmacologic and non-pharmacologic treatments, as well as engaging in discussions regarding care goals with both patients and their families. Achieving an enhancement in the quality of life for these children requires the implementation of an aggressive approach toward the management of their symptoms.

## 6.3 Managing Common Respiratory Symptom in Pediatrics

### 6.3.1 Introduction

Respiratory difficulties are prevalent and distressing and can persist for extended periods. They affect approximately 25.6% of pediatric patients with genetic, metabolic, or neurological conditions, which tend to worsen with time. Parents of children experiencing severe cardiovascular issues frequently report that respiratory distress in the terminal stage of life is often associated with considerable or significant pain, with a correlation noted in 77% of pediatric patients younger than 2 years and 62% of those aged 2 years or older [144].

### 6.3.2 Dyspnea

One of the most common symptoms that parents who are involved in their child's care report is shortness of breath, or dyspnea, which is the medical term for the uncomfortable feeling of difficulty breathing. It's been noted in 24% of child in the last 3 days of their lives, ranking second only to pain as the most frequent symptom. Among child with cancer, dyspnea affects 49% in the last month of life and is deliberately extreme in 29.4% of cases [145]. Since shortness of breath is a subjective feeling, the only way to accurately measure it is through the child's own report, which can be a challenge in situations where many children are unable to report or have not learned to describe their symptoms. There is a scale designed for the assessment of dyspnea in children, but it might not always be accurate or easy to use for some groups of patients [145].

#### 6.3.2.1 Management of Dyspnea

Ease of approach in managing dyspnea is the key, and it can start while focusing on treating the symptoms or addressing the cause of dyspnea. Both anxiety and dyspnea can intensify each other.

- Comprehensive explanation of potential causes accompanied by ongoing reassurance for both the child and their family.
- Positioning the child upright, allowing them to lean forward or propping the head of the bed up to improve ease of breathing.
- Utilizing natural ventilation through opened windows or artificial ventilation such as electric or manual fans to ensure air circulation and movement toward the child's breathing zone.
- Applying a cold compress to the child's forehead to alleviate discomfort.
- Employing methods of distraction tailored to the child's age group, including play, music therapy, and respiratory exercises.
- In instances involving older children, investigating potential psychological causes of dyspnea and offering reassurance and supportive counseling as needed.
- Ensuring oral hygiene to combat the effects of dry mouth caused by mouth breathing.
- For episodes of dyspnea related to anxiety and recurring in nature, consultation with additional team members, such as social workers, counselors, or psychologists, to provide further counseling may be beneficial.

#### 6.3.2.2 Pharmacological Measures

- The efficacy of opioid use in mitigating symptom relief from difficulty in breathing in adults has been substantiated through various research studies. As a result, opioid medications frequently serve as the initial line of treatment in pediatric patients [146].
- For severe shortness of breath, the administration of morphine might be warranted. This is

attributed to its dual role in alleviating both anxiety and pain. Should the patient be not on an opioid regimen, the initial dose of morphine should be reduced to one-third of the standard starting dose. Conversely, for patients already prescribed morphine, a dose increment of half should be considered.

- Bronchodilators, coupled with oxygen therapy, may prove beneficial in the presence of bronchospasm symptoms.
- The use of saline nebulizers could prove advantageous in facilitating the thinning of secretions and maintaining the moistness of airways.
- In instances involving fluid retention and accompanying shortness of breath, particularly in pediatric cases linked to pulmonary edema or congestive heart failure, diuretics may offer considerable support.
- Anxiety relief may be achieved through the administration of anxiolytics, such as benzodiazepines, including diazepam (Valium) and lorazepam (Ativan). This approach is particularly effective when there is an anxiety-induced component to the patient's respiratory distress.
- In situations where a patient experiences brief, severe shortness of breath but remains adequately oxygenated, the administration of oxygen therapy may not directly alleviate the symptom.

### 6.3.3 Cough

In managing children who need palliative care, the primary causes of cough typically include infectious agents (whether acute or chronic), aspiration (especially in cases where there is an impairment in swallowing function), gastroesophageal reflux, and, albeit rarely, malignancy. The efficacy of a cough depends on the strength of the mucous membrane and the capability to generate sufficient airway velocity. A failure to develop an effective cough can result in chronic and troubling coughing episodes, adversely influencing sleep quality and exacerbating symptoms such as nausea, pain, and dyspnea [147].

#### 6.3.3.1 Management of Cough

- Reducing the amount of food or starting continuous feeding can be a good way to address gastrointestinal reflux.
- For children experiencing difficulty swallowing, a reduction in cough associated with aspiration may be achieved through modifications in feeding techniques or a transition from oral to nasogastric tube feeding routes.
- Managing excessive secretions accumulating in the oropharynx can be facilitated through the implementation of postural drainage, suctioning, and physiotherapy.
- If a tumor mass is blocking the airway, therapies aimed at reducing the tumor mass's size should also be taken into account.
- Efficient chest physiotherapy is imperative for children who are facing heightened viscosity of secretions and/or an inability to effectively clear their airways, which often results from muscle weakness.

### 6.3.4 Hemoptysis

Hemoptysis, defined as the expectoration of blood, is often encountered in pediatric patients undergoing palliative care, especially among those diagnosed with hematological malignancies, Coagulation disorders, which may arise from numerous factors such as disseminated intravascular coagulation and respiratory infections, can cause considerable distress for both the child and their parents. The mere presence of even a minimal quantity of blood-stained sputum can heighten concerns regarding the potential for a more serious and life-threatening hemorrhage [148].

#### 6.3.4.1 Management of Hemoptysis

- It is advisable to consider routine platelet transfusions for pediatric patients presenting with thrombocytopenia, despite the considerable burden associated with frequent hospital visits potentially overshadowing any potential advantages [149].

- Non-medical interventions encompass repositioning, keeping child calm and the initiation of postural drainage. Additionally, suctioning, though generally providing only short-term benefits, might also prove beneficial.
- Anticholinergic medications, primarily comprising hyoscine hydrobromide or glycopyrronium, are frequently used.

### 6.3.5 Summary

In pediatric, respiratory symptoms in the terminal phase of life are prevalent, cause significant distress, and exert a profound influence on the well-being of parents. There is a critical need for a carefully designed, interdisciplinary pediatric approach to demonstrate the efficacy of commonly used interventions and their influence on the quality of life for both the child and their family. Given the limited availability of pediatric evidence, it is necessary to address the treatment of each child on an individual basis, primarily drawing upon established best practices from adult studies. The treatment regimen should be tailored to the observed individual benefit of each child.

## 6.4 Managing Psychological Symptoms in Pediatric Palliative Care

### 6.4.1 Introduction

Palliative care extends beyond managing symptoms; it also encompasses addressing the wider impact of illness, death, and grief on children and their families. This is particularly significant because it recognizes that physical, profound, and spiritual needs cannot be addressed in isolation, as each facet influences the other. For instance, a child's pain may lead to increased anxiety in parents, and familial stress can complicate the management of pain.

Children with serious medical conditions are more prone to developing a range of mental and physical health symptoms, including depression, anxiety, pain, nausea/vomiting, fatigue, delirium, and difficulty breathing [150]. Research indicates a bidirectional relationship between physical illness and psychosocial distress, suggesting that psychosocial distress can worsen physical health symptoms (such as pain intensifying with heightened anxiety) and vice versa.

The provision of palliative care can also give rise to various psychological and emotional challenges in children, such as distress, depression, anxiety, and social isolation. There is also an increased risk for depression, anxiety, post-traumatic stress disorder, and grief [151]. When caregivers do not openly discuss their child's impending death, they may encounter difficulties in inter-professional communication among healthcare providers, divergent treatment goals between staff and the child, fears and uncertainties regarding the child's prognosis, and regret.

Psychological assessment in pediatric palliative care presents a unique challenge as there are no specific tools designed for this population. Nevertheless, there exist tools that encompass a wide range of domains, such as the PedsQL and PROMIS instruments. The PedsQL is a concise assessment tool that evaluates the health-related quality of life of children and young individuals. The completion of this task involves the participation of both parents via the intermediary report and the child or young person through self-reporting. The measure is composed of 23 items, which are divided into 4 domains: physical health, psychological well-being, social functioning, and general health.

1. Physical health (eight items).
2. Psychological well-being (five items).
3. Social functioning (five items).
4. School functioning (five items).

Following instruction from a credentialed administrator, the Pediatric Quality of Life Inventory (PedsQL) can be independently administered by parents, children, and adolescents between the ages of 8 and 18 years within approximately 5 min. It is recommended that clinicians manage the inventory for younger individuals, particularly in special situations, such as when all items and instructions are read aloud to the child or adolescent. Before consulting with a physician or other healthcare professional, it is advisable for respondents to complete the inventory prior to filling out any other health-related data forms. Additionally, guidelines for the administration of the PedsQL inventory are accessible via the Internet.

- PedsQL 8–12 years for child (self-reported).
- PedsQL 8–12 years for parent (parent-reported).

### 6.4.2 Patient-Reported Outcomes Measurement Information System (PROMIS) Instrument

The instruments known as the Pediatric and Parent Proxy Profile consist of a set of concise forms. Each form includes a single item that assesses pain intensity, along with a specific number of items from six different PROMIS domains: depressive symptoms, anxiety, physical function and mobility, pain interference, fatigue, and peer relationships. Among children, the preferred approach for evaluating outcomes is typically through the process of self-report. However, in instances where a child is deemed too young, exhibits cognitive difficulties, or is unable to take the test due to illness, parents are relied upon to provide proxy reports on their child's behalf. It is important to recognize that scores derived from both parent proxy reports and self-report measures may not align perfectly. This discrepancy is attributed to the distinct perspectives these two methods offer, which could potentially influence healthcare utilization, risk factors, or the quality of care.

Thus, a comprehensive assessment that considers both the child's and the parent's viewpoints is highly recommended. Providers should carefully evaluate the child's ability to understand and accurately respond to questions posed, thereby facilitating the decision between the use of the Pediatric Self-Report Profile and the Parent Proxy Profile. Should there be any uncertainty, the Proxy Profile may be considered as an alternative.

### 6.4.3 Anxiety

Anxiety is a state of worry or unease that is frequently linked to an upcoming event that is feared or uncertain. Even if it is not pathologic, anxiety can have a negative impact on a child's quality of life and be under-recognized in seriously ill children, especially in the early stages following a diagnosis [152].

#### 6.4.3.1 Causes of Anxiety

Physical symptoms like dyspnea, nausea, and pain—both acute and chronic—often directly cause acute anxiety in patients of all ages. Anxiety can be brought on by adverse effects of invasive procedures like intravenous access, chemotherapy, and surgery, as well as drugs like corticosteroids that are frequently prescribed to seriously ill patients. Anxiety can also be brought on or exacerbated by individual medical conditions and psychiatric disorders that are co-occurring.

#### 6.4.3.2 Assessment of Anxiety

The reliability and validity of the following assessment scales have been demonstrated in the pediatric age group: Memorial Symptom Assessment Scale (MSAS), Patient-Reported Outcomes Measurement Information System (PROMIS), and Screen for Child Anxiety Related Emotional Disorders (SCARED). These tools/scales can be used to assess anxiety in the pediatric population [153–155].

#### 6.4.3.3 Management of Anxiety

- Involvement of multidisciplinary team that includes social workers, therapists, child care specialists, spiritual healers, etc.
- Counseling.
- Mild anxiolytic in moderate to severe anxiety [156].

### 6.4.4 Depression

Children and teenagers who are terminally ill or have long-term medical conditions are more likely to experience depression. Parents must be aware of this and watch for any indications that their child is becoming depressed. This will incorporate the child turning out to be peaceful and removed or peevish. Treatments that work are out there, just like they are for adults. However, treatments must be tailored precisely and typically involve the entire family.

#### 6.4.4.1 Management of Depression

Psychological counseling always enhances the child's autonomy and strength to make decisions. Psychologist play a significant role in providing psychotherapy (counseling), and other interventions can help children and adolescents feel more confident, build and sustain healthy relationships, and reduce symptoms. If child condtion will not get improved using psychotherapy, a supportive pharmacological intervention therapy using medication such as anti-depressents will be useful.

### 6.4.5 Insomnia

At some point, children who have been diagnosed with a serious illness have trouble sleeping. This could be as a result of general anxiety, treatment-related anxiety, or worries about the future. As a matter of fact, getting to rest might be the most troublesome aspect.

#### 6.4.5.1 Measures to Overcome Sleeping Issues

- Make an effort to establish a regular bedtime routine and fall asleep at the same time each night.
- Try to provide warm milk before going to bed.
- Play a favorite music rather than tossing and turning in bed.
- Tell the favorite story before the sleep.

### 6.4.6 Psychological Interventions

The primary objective of psychological interventions is to diminish the burden of symptoms. This can be achieved through various methods, including cognitive-behavioral therapy, coping techniques, and relaxation therapy. However, acceptance and mindfulness-based therapy might be less effective for pediatric patients facing terminal illnesses. In such cases, the active involvement of family members and collaborative communication between the child/parent and the multidisciplinary team on the plan of care and the treatment preferences are highly recommended.

#### 6.4.6.1 Management of Common Psychological Issues

- Consider the child's preferences for support.
- Give the child free reign.
- When possible, let the child make choices.
- As much as possible, respond truthfully to inquiries.
- Respond to the request effectively.
- Be careful not to overwhelm the child with excess of information that they do not want.
- It's possible that children only require a small amount of information at a time.
- While drawing or doing another activity, children might find it easier to talk.
- Emotions can be released through play, creative writing, music, and other creative endeavors.
- Comfort with physical contact.

### 6.4.7 Summary

Children may change care settings, increasing care complexity. To avoid overwhelming the family, careful coordination is essential. As a result of some staff members' erroneous assumption that others have assumed responsibility for a particular task, there is also the possibility that families will receive inadequate support. Appointing a "key worker" or "case manager" may be beneficial in situations where a large number of services are involved. This individual might be an overall professional, pediatrician, nurture, or united well-being specialist.

## 6.5 Management of Neurological Symptoms in Palliative Care

In settings dedicated to palliative care, neurological symptoms can arise from a multitude of causes, such as primary and metastatic cancers, neurodegenerative disease, and the medication-associated adverse drug reactions. The approach to management must consider the specific condition causing the symptoms, as well as the precise location of any identified lesions. In numerous instances, definitive treatment options may not be available, yet it is often possible to effectively manage the symptoms.

Cancer within the nervous system ranks as the second most prevalent cancer in children, with more often encountered types including astrocytoma and medulloblastomas. Additionally, brain tumors can manifest as metastases from other types of cancer, such as lymphomas. The manifestation of neurological symptoms is highly dependent on the nature and position of the tumor within the central nervous system.

### 6.5.1 Myoclonus

Myoclonus refers to the transient and sporadic contractions that can involve the entire muscle or a portion of it. These contractions may arise from various factors, including immobility, pain, and other forms of sensory stimulants. Earlier, it is also notified as a side effect of opioid use, with a particular association with pethidine, and its prevalence tends to increase among individuals with renal impairment [157].

Treatment Considerations for Myoclonus

- Treatment options for myoclonus are not always required, especially if the symptoms do not adversely affect the patient. In instances where treatment is deemed necessary, measures can include reducing the opioid dosage, altering the administration route, or transitioning to an alternative medication.
- Benzodiazepines are effective in managing myoclonus, with specific recommendations ranging from oral doses of 0.05–0.1 mg/kg every 4–6 h.
- A maximum of 5 mg per dose for oral diazepam and oral or sublingual clonazepam doses of 0.01 mg/kg every 8–12 h.
- Midazolam can also be administered continuously via SC or IV infusion for effective seizure management, at rates between 8 and 30 micrograms/kg/hour.

### 6.5.2 Muscle Spasm

Muscle spasm, also known as pediatric myoclonus, is the term for a child's rapid, jerking muscle movements. The child has no control over these uncontrollable movements. It is characterized by an excruciating, involuntary contraction of the skeletal muscle, usually involving the flexor group. This condition frequently manifests as a symptom when upper motor neuron lesions are present.

Treatment strategies for muscle spasm include:

- Baclofen: Administer 0.5 mg/kg/day, dose with increments of 0.5 mg in every 3–4 days, aiming to reach an optimum dosage of 0.6 mg/kg over the course of 8 h, if tolerated. Baclofen may also be administered intrathecally for effectiveness.
- Dantrolene: This medication is administered at a recommended dose range of 0.1–0.3 mg/kg between 1 and 4 h as needed, up to a maximum dosage of 0.6 mg/kg in 8 h.
- Diazepam IV: Administration via oral route is not recommended for diazepam in this case. Instead, it should be used via intravenous route at a dosage of 0.1–0.3 mg/kg every

1–4 h, as necessary, with a maximum dosage of 0.6 mg/kg in the span of 8 h.
- Oral Route: An oral dosage given in every 8–12 h range of 0.05–0.3 mg/kg [158].

### 6.5.3 Delirium

Children and adolescents can suffer from delirium, a dangerous illness marked by profound disorientation and behavioral abnormalities. It is a clinical emergency that needs to be handled right away. Upon onset, symptoms may present as acute or subacute, and there may be discernible fluctuations in symptoms observed over the course of the day.

The approach to managing delirium encompasses several strategies:

- Addressing the root cause, if feasible (often, a precise cause cannot be determined, and in some cases, death may be inevitable).
- Treatment of specific medical conditions or substances.
- Management of metabolic imbalances.
- Prevention and treatment of dehydration.
- Mitigation of factors that aggravate the condition, including severe pain, urinary retention, hypoxia, medication interactions, and fear.
- Creating an environment for care that is quiet and secure.
- Providing sedation as necessary.
- Pharmacological interventions includes administration of medication such as haloperidol 0.01-0.1 mg/kg orally or via intravenous route in 8 hourly, with a recommended dose upto 2 mg.
- Alternatively, clonazepam 0.01 mg/kg sublingual every 8–12 h, with a dose of 2 mg, may be administered. The choice of medication and dosage is adjusted based on the patient's response [159].

### 6.5.4 Seizure

Management of seizures in newborns warrants particular attention. Similar to their pediatric counterparts, the preferred method of administering medications to neonates is through oral, oro-gastric, or nasogastric routes. However, it is important to note that due to variations in pharmacokinetics, medication choices and dosages are distinct from those employed in older children. The drug phenobarbitone is notably favored for its efficacy in managing seizures in newborns [160].

### 6.5.5 Pharmacological Management

- Phenobarbitone: Initial dose—0.20 mg/kg intravenous loading dose, which may be divided into two equal parts. Subsequent dose: 0.05 mg/kg/day intravenous (IV) and oral maintenance dose.
- Phenytoin: Initial dose—0.20 mg/kg, loading dose via intravenous, followed by 0.04 mg/kg/day oral maintenance dose.
- Clonazepam: Initial dose—0.25 mg/kg intravenous (IV) loading dose (for infants not on mechanical ventilation; 0.1–0.2 mg/kg/day maintenance dose via oral route is acceptable). Subsequent dose: 0.01–0.03 mg/kg/day oral maintenance dose.
- In case an infant exhibits signs of drowsiness or fails to respond to the anticonvulsant regimen, cessation of anticonvulsant therapy should be considered. Subsequent seizures, if they occur, should be addressed using clonazepam [161].

**In children with 6 months of age or older:**

Children who are diagnosed with primary or metastatic brain tumors, genetic abnormalities, or metabolic dysfunctions may experience a heightened susceptibility to seizures. Such occurrences can be emotionally challenging for family members, and it is often beneficial for parents to acquire comprehensive information regarding the management and treatment of seizures [162].

- The administration of diazepam, in doses ranging from 0.3 to 0.5 mg rectally, has been found to be efficacious.
- As an alternative anticonvulsant, midazolam can also be employed. This parenteral medica-

tion may be given either directly via buccal route or by intranasal route, with a dosage ranging from 0.3 to 0.5 mg/kg (with a maximum dose of 10 mg).
- In instances where a child is not able to tolerate administrations of anticonvulsants either oral or rectal route, midazolam may be administered intravenously or subcutaneously.
- In management of emergency seizures, the initial dosage is set at 0.15 mg/kg intravenously or subcutaneously on the scene, followed by a dosage increment of 2 micrograms/kg/min, increased by the same increments, until the cessation of seizures is observed, with a maximum rate not exceeding 24 micrograms/kg/min.

### 6.5.6 Summary

Children with complex medical conditions frequently exhibit neurological symptoms, which pose significant challenges for accurate assessment and treatment. Identifying and differentiating between various neurological symptoms necessitates an in-depth medical history and thorough verification of all possible causative factors. It is essential to meticulously investigate and address pain, be it nociceptive or neuropathic in nature. Treatment strategies encompass both non-pharmacological therapies and pharmaceutical interventions, being considered in cases of severe intractability. The management of such children is strongly advocated for through collaborative, interdisciplinary efforts.

## 6.6 Managing Skin-Associated Symptoms Among Children

### 6.6.1 Introduction

The prevalence of skin diseases is notably higher among patients receiving palliative care, a group characterized by an immunosuppressed condition and reduced mobility. Research supports the observation that individuals within this category are more likely to develop decubitus ulcers or experience worsening of pre-existing ulcers. Common dermatological diagnoses in these patients include dermatitis, xerosis, and pruritus.

### 6.6.2 Pruritus

Pruritus is defined as an unpleasant sensation on the skin that manifests as a desire to scratch. It is often synonymous with the term "itchiness." The underlying causes of pruritus encompass a variety of factors, including dry skin (known as xerosis), dermatitis (which is characterized by skin inflammation), scabies (a mite infestation), chickenpox, obstructive jaundice, and adverse reactions to certain medications. In the case of a child presenting with generalized itchiness and a persistent urge to rub their nose, it is indicative that opioids may be a primary culprit. This condition may prove transient, lasting for a few days, but alternative opioids may need to be considered if the itchiness persists [163].

#### 6.6.2.1 Assessment of Pruritus

Pruritus is the subjective feeling of itching that causes rubbing or scratching, which can cause damage to the skin. A comprehensive skin examination, a review of the child's exposure history, and occasionally laboratory testing are required to evaluate pruritus in children. The Itching Severity Scale (ISS), Visual Analogue Scale (VAS), Numerical Scale, and Verbal Scale are the instruments used to measure the intensity of itching. A clinical examination is also pivotal in assessing pruritus. This involves assessing for dryness of skin, inflammation of skin (dermatitis), jaundice, skin rashes, and the presence of chronic conditions like psoriasis or eczema.

#### 6.6.2.2 Non-pharmacological Measures

- To alleviate pruritus, it is recommended to moisturize the skin regularly using emollient-based products (emollients, lotions, creams), as dry skin is a common cause of itchiness.
- It is advised to avoid the use of lanolin-based products due to the risk of causing allergic reactions.
- Eliminating possible allergens, including scented items, and irritants like rough bedding is advantageous.

- Furthermore, the adoption of gentle soaps in minimal quantities, the avoidance of hot water during bathing or showering, the exclusion of abrasive materials like washcloths and sponges, and the method of gently patting the skin dry instead of vigorously rubbing it can aid in alleviating symptoms.
- Distraction strategies, such as music therapy, recreational activities, and bubble blowing exercises, have proven successful in managing symptoms of itchiness.

#### 6.6.2.3 Pharmacological Measures

- When managing severe itchiness or individual lesions, the application of topical ointments or creams with antipruritic property, such as urea, 1% Mentholatum, at regular interval daily is advisable.
- Topical application of steroids may also be beneficial in severe cases or for the treatment of individual lesions, with the starting concentration typically being hydrocortisone 1%.
- The dosage strength may need to be increased as required.
- Sedating with oral antihistamines for use at night, such as chlorpheniramine (Allergex), is considered, with the exception of itch induced by morphine, in which case, ondansetron is recommended [164].

### 6.6.3 Pressure Ulcer

A pressure sore, also referred to as a bed sore or pressure ulcer, emerges as a condition characterized by skin and underlying tissue damage, a consequence of diminished blood flow that consequently deprives the tissues of vital oxygen and nutrients. Infants and children, especially those afflicted with severe illnesses or constrained mobility, are notably susceptible to the onset of these ulcers. Various medical devices, including cervical collars, oxygen cylinders, nasogastric tubes, and catheters, may also play a role in the development of pressure ulcers.

#### 6.6.3.1 Risk Groups for Pressure Ulcer

- Newborn infants immobilized or connected to medical devices like CPAP prongs.
- Children suffering from neurological conditions that include cerebral palsy, spina bifida, or other life-limiting illnesses.
- Young individuals, including both children and adolescents, who are confined to bed rest, suffer from malnutrition, or are characterized by obesity.

#### 6.6.3.2 Causes of Pressure Ulcer

1. **Pressure onto the skin:** This phenomenon occurs when the body's weight exerts pressure on the skin or when external objects or medical devices, such as wheelchairs, urinary catheter tubing, gastrostomy or nasogastric tubes, splints, body braces, intravenous lines, saturation probes, or plaster casts, come into contact with the skin.
2. **Due to friction:** Friction is initiated when the skin is subjected to repeated pulling or rubbing against a surface, including beds, bedding, or other equipment. This may result from a child sliding down a bed or chair or due to improper handling and movement techniques.
3. **Moisture:** Prolonged moisture on the skin elevates its susceptibility to degradation, thereby increasing the risk of developing pressure ulcers. Children who are incontinent and infants left unattended in wet diapers are particularly vulnerable.
4. **History of skin damage:** Children or infants who have previously experienced a pressure ulcer are at a higher risk of developing new ones [165].

#### 6.6.3.3 Strategies to Prevent Pressure Sores

**To prevent pressure sores, the following strategies can be implemented:**

- Implement a schedule for turning the child every 2–4 h, whenever feasible.

- Utilize specialized equipment like air mattresses, air rings, and cushions to distribute pressure more evenly across the body.
- Position the head of a newborn or a child attached to a ventilator when turning them.
- Conduct regular inspections by assessing pressure point area of the skin each time the child is turned.
- Ensure that any therapeutic devices in contact with the child's skin do not exert unnecessary pressure, including nasogastric tubes, nasal cannula, and splints.
- Make sure that the skin is washed and dried regularly, including bed baths for patients who are bedridden.
- Prevent the damage of the skin by lifting the child rather than dragging or restraining them.
- Educate and provide advice to the child's family members about assessing early signs of pressure injury and the necessary steps to reduce their formation in home care setting.
- Always make sure that the bed linen remains dry and wrinkle-free and folds.
- Keep the area around the diaper area clean and dry, with frequent changes in diapers [166].

**A variety of strategies are employed in the treatment of pressure ulcers:**

- Utilization of cushions to bolster joints plays a pivotal role, facilitating relaxation and preventing excessive joint overstretching.
- The elimination of necrotic tissue is crucial: Surgical debridement involves the use of scissors or a scalpel. The process of autolytic debridement uses the body's natural enzymes to remove dead tissue from a wound. Children's pressure ulcers can be treated with it, particularly if surgical debridement is not an option. A hydrocolloid dressing or wound gel can be used to create a moist wound environment for autolytic debridement.
- Bleeding can be managed by cauterization, applying gauze saturated with a 1:1000 solution of epinephrine, using non-adhesive dressings, applying topical low-dose (100 units/ml) epinephrine solution, and carefully removing dressings moistened first with warmed normal saline and use thromboplastin or silver nitrate (0·5–1%).
- Addressing infection: Irrigation of the wound with warm, sterile saline or continuous water flow is recommended. The application of systemic and topical antibiotics is essential.
- Selection of dressings: Maintaining an optimal moisture balance is achieved through the use of hydrogel dressing and films. To enhance moisture levels, hydrogels are employed. To protect the integrity of the wound surface, contact layers are necessary, such as impregnated gauze (Jelonet) or Bactigras. Antimicrobial properties are ensured with the application of glycerine, ichthammol, silver sulfadiazine cream, activated charcoal, and silver-containing dressings.

### 6.6.4 Managing Malodorous Fungating Wounds in Pediatric

This complex condition predominantly presents itself in young individuals, with a higher prevalence observed in those with more advanced primary skin cancers, skin metastases, or malignancies that extend into the bone, muscle, or connective tissues. This condition arises when the tumor exhibits a rapid increase in its growth through the skin, leading to the formation of ulcers and necrosis. The term "fungating wound" characterizes the distinctive appearance of the affected skin, which exhibits features that mimic those of a fungus [167].

#### 6.6.4.1 Determining the Origin of the Malodor

The malodor (bad smell) emanates due to the presence of anaerobic bacteria in the necrotic tissue of the fungating wound.

#### 6.6.4.2 Assessment of Malodorous Fungating Wound in a Child

A thorough assessment of the child includes the following elements:

- The nutritional status of the child.
- Medications being administered.
- A history of indication of chemotherapy or radiation therapy.
- A thorough clinical evaluation and assessment of the wound location, appearance, size, odor, presence of exudates, and the condition of the nearby skin.
- Demonstrated systemic manifestations of infection.

#### 6.6.4.3 Management Strategies for Fungating Malodorous Wounds

- The management strategies involve the active participation of the child in decision-making processes, such as determining the timing of dressing changes and the presence of spectators.
- Preparatory measures should include explaining how to clean the wound and employing distraction methods, such as telling a story or blowing bubbles.
- The procedure done using aseptic techniques, during cleaning, irrigation, and wound debridement (the removal of dead tissue), significantly reduces the infection and, consequently, the malodor.
- Additionally, the application of activated charcoal to the wound dressing can help absorb odors.
- The significance of managing malodor cannot be overemphasized, given its critical role in the psychological welfare of the child and their relatives.
- For pain, a procedural dose, administered 30 min prior to the wound cleaning and dressing, is particularly recommended [168].

#### 6.6.4.4 Specific Measures for Controlling the Malodor

- Application of metronidazole cream during each dressing change.
- A compounding formula for the cream can be prepared by dissolving 1 tub of aqueous cream with 40 tablets of metronidazole (Flagyl) in 400 mg doses and adding morphine powder 10 mg.
- Metronidazole solution can be formulated by dissolving 13 tablets of metronidazole (Flagyl) in 400 mg doses in 2 L of saline solution. The solution should be used for cleaning and irrigation of the wound gently.
- Environmental measures to manage the malodor include utilizing natural ventilation through open windows and doors whenever feasible.
- The avoidance of air fresheners or perfumes as they may not effectively minimize the malodor and could potentially associate their fragrance with the wound odor.

### 6.6.5 Summary

Children under palliative care are at an increased risk of developing decubitus ulcers and cutaneous infections. The aggressive management of systemic symptoms can inadvertently exacerbate skin conditions. It is crucial, therefore, to take into account dermatological conditions when devising a plan to optimize skin care in this specific patient population.

# 7 End-of-Life Care of Pediatric with Advanced Illness

## 7.1 End-of-Life Care of Pediatric

A comprehensive approach to the frequently complex physical, social, psychological, and spiritual needs of a child in end-of-life care who has a progressive and advanced illness, as well as assistance with advance care planning, are necessary for the family. To meet these needs, a pediatric palliative care team with a variety of skills and abilities is unavoidably needed. Pediatric end-of-life care, the importance of communication, advanced medical directives, the role of a multidisciplinary team, and caregivers are all covered in this chapter. Advanced care planning to assist the families is covered, along with the important ethical concerns for the child with a terminal illness.

### 7.1.1 Communication

In the context of a terminally ill child, effective communication becomes of utmost importance. Engaging in end-of-life discussions with caregivers is crucial to avoid the pursuit of aggressive, futile medical interventions, subpar quality of life, or heightened challenges in coping with bereavement [170].

Using collaborative communication techniques, which include but are not restricted to resolving possible misunderstandings, setting goals together, and recognizing, honoring, and reacting to different forms of understanding and compassion [171].

#### 7.1.1.1 Measures to Enhance Communication

- Help parents to acknowledge and amend unrealistic anticipations.
- It is imperative to meticulously record all forms of communication.
- Encourage dialogue among family members, especially with adolescents, to facilitate the sharing of emotions and to designate quality family time.
- Permit a terminally ill child to engage in discussions with the treatment team, addressing their fears and inquiries in an appropriate context.
- Numerous children possess an innate awareness of their impending death and may utilize symbolic expressions to articulate this understanding.
- Emphasize the principles of honesty, empathy, and the reassurance of efforts to ensure a pain-free transition [172].

#### 7.1.1.2 Ethical Considerations in Pediatric Palliative Care

In the realm of pediatric medical decision-making, it is a standard protocol for healthcare professionals to transfer decision-making authority to the parent or caregiver overseeing the child. This practice is often observed while equipping


N. Javadi-Pashaki et al., *Interdisciplinary Pediatric Palliative Care*,
https://doi.org/10.1007/978-981-97-9587-1_7

families with detailed information regarding the progression of the child's condition, the proposed treatments, and the anticipated prognosis [173].

The foundational ethical principles guiding advance care planning mirror those in various healthcare situations, including pediatric palliative care. These principles include respect for autonomy, beneficence, and non-maleficence. All therapeutic interventions should be evaluated in terms of their anticipated benefits versus potential burdens. Consequently, the treatment should only be administered when the benefits significantly outweigh the burdens. This poses a considerable challenge, as it necessitates the precise forecasting of benefits and drawbacks within the complex environments characterized by uncertainty and a range of values [174].

#### 7.1.1.3 Doctrine of Double Effect

The doctrine of double effect stipulates that aim of alleviating suffering is permissible, provided that any potential risks or adverse consequences, such as a reduction in survival duration, are inadvertently caused by the healthcare professional. The choice to commence or cease resuscitative efforts, which includes all measures intended to preserve and support cardiovascular, respiratory, and metabolic activities, ultimately rests with the parents. This decision ought to be made prior to the occurrence of any acute event. Orders designating a patient as unresponsive should be meticulously drafted and executed by the parents prior to such events.

### 7.1.2 Euthanasia

Euthanasia refers to the intentional and painless termination of life for an individual suffering from a terminal illness that is incurable, destined to lead to death. Allowing for the natural death of a person distinctively differs from euthanasia, both in intention, action, and the professional duty involved. The intention of euthanasia is to precipitously induce death, whereas the purpose of discontinuing life-sustaining treatment is to end a process that is inherently unavoidable. Euthanasia is still prohibited in Australia and New Zealand, even after much discussion, but it is legal in the Netherlands and Belgium for both active and passive euthanasia. Passive euthanasia is permitted in India, England, and the United States.

In certain circumstances, parents and other family members may broach the topic of euthanasia with their loved ones, either directly or indirectly. While it is appropriate to clarify the legal stance, it is paramount to understand the true concerns of the parents and their comprehension of euthanasia. Often, the primary concerns of the parents are centered around the suffering of their child and can be adequately addressed through high-quality palliative care. Furthermore, it's not uncommon for parents' views on euthanasia to diverge from the conventional medical perspective, which may include apprehensions about the necessity for resuscitation and the constraints on pain relief due to the dual effect of analgesics [30, 175].

#### 7.1.2.1 Location of End-of-Life Care

The decision regarding the suitable placement of end-of-life care for a terminally ill child depends on a multitude of elements. These factors encompass the family's choice, the living conditions of the child's household, the individual's religious or spiritual convictions, and the financial constraints.

This decision should be entered into with the involvement of the child, if their maturity and comprehension permit, alongside family members. The ultimate goal is to ensure the child's final stages of life are characterized by comfort and security. Respecting the child's wishes, the comfort of familiar surroundings, and the parental aspiration to serve as the primary caregiver are among the factors influencing the preference for the hospital as the setting for the child's demise. This preference is largely driven by trust in the personnel of the hospital, the logistical convenience of the facility, and the perceived safety of the hospital environment [176].

**The potential care settings include:**

- Hospice care, which focuses on providing comfort, support, and medical management of symptoms.
- In-patient care, which is deemed necessary if the child requires continuous consistent medical attention.

- Home-based care, which involves supplying the family with the necessary medications for managing pain and other symptoms, in collaboration with a nearby physician.

#### 7.1.2.2 Management of Symptoms

A significant number of children progressing toward the end of life experience severe physical symptoms spanning from weeks to months prior to death. These symptoms may include but are not limited to pain, shortness of breath, fever, and bleeding. Patients who exhibit more pronounced symptoms often seek care at a higher-level tertiary care facility or return to their initial healthcare institution for management. It is imperative to exercise caution in the administration of medications due to the potential for interactions among multiple drugs, malnutrition, hypoalbuminemia (low levels of albumin), and reduced liver and kidney function among other factors.

### 7.1.3 Pain

It is frequently noted that there is often an escalation in pain severity toward the final stages of a child's life. Nonetheless, it is crucial to recognize that while some children may experience significant suffering before passing away, there are instances where certain children will succumb to death without having endured extensive pain. The suffering endured at the terminal end of a child's life manifests as a multifaceted amalgamation of physical, psychological, social, spiritual, and additional factors [177].

#### 7.1.3.1 Strategy for Managing Pain

- The implementation of predefined management strategies, in conjunction with the availability of rapid-acting opioids, enables the successful management of the majority of pediatric patients. Typically, this can be achieved through the administration of morphine elixir, which is to be given every 4 hours, and its dosage is incrementally increased by 30–50% as required.
- In situations where a child cannot swallow or access through a gastrostomy or nasogastric tube is not feasible, morphine can be given orally or rectal.
- In instances where facilities allow, the utilization of syringe drivers has been demonstrated to be highly efficacious.

#### 7.1.3.2 The Death Rattle

The occurrence of the death rattle is frequently witnessed in the later stages of a patient's ailment and can cause significant distress to the attending family members. It is imperative that they are adequately informed and prepared for such events. The production of this unique sound is a result of the movement of loudly secreted fluids within the child's airways, as their ability to effectively cough or swallow these secretions diminishes. It is noteworthy that this phenomenon is more inclined to manifest as the child's level of consciousness decreases. Consequently, it should not be solely regarded as a cause of distress for the child.

#### 7.1.3.3 Management Strategies

The management of the death rattle should be implemented with the following strategies in mind:

- Correct positioning of the child's head to facilitate the drainage of secretions.
- Should it be associated with dyspnea, administration of opioids and/or benzodiazepines may be warranted.
- Employing either subcutaneous or transdermal hyoscine therapy could be beneficial.
- The application of gentle suction should be employed [178].

### 7.1.4 Dyspnea

When a child shows symptoms of dyspnea, it is critical to determine whether the symptom is caused by a treatable condition, such as asthma or heart failure. Giving a small dose of opioids or benzodiazepines may help in situations where breathing difficulties are only a symptom of an incurable illness. In cases where the difficulty of breathing is solely a manifestation of an incurable disease, the administration of a low dosage of opioids or benzodiazepines may prove beneficial [179].

#### 7.1.4.1 Nutrition and Hydration

Children facing advanced or terminal illnesses often cease their intake of food and fluids when they become unable to digest them. This condition, known as anorexia, coupled with a dislike of food, can significantly distress family members.

Managing this situation involves recognizing and respecting the natural instinct to nourish a child. It also entails providing counseling to parents or caregivers to alleviate their anxiety. Mandating the consumption of food or fluids may result in aspiration, and the initiation of artificial nutrition and hydration does not automatically extend the child's lifespan and enhance their quality of life, strength, or activity levels. It is important to understand that refraining from hydration does not result in suffering if the child is at ease or unconscious [180].

Encouraging alternative methods for family members to maintain their connection and provide care, such as gentle massage, is also crucial. Additionally, proper mouth care, including moisturizing the mouth with water and protecting the lips from dryness, is essential. It is important to note that a considerable proportion of terminally ill patients do not suffer from hunger. However, among those who do experience hunger, providing them with modest amounts of food and fluids in response to their requests can effectively manage their hunger.

#### 7.1.4.2 Advantages of Dehydration during the Terminal Phase

- Diminished production of respiratory secretions.
- Significantly mitigated discomfort including nausea, vomiting, abdominal bloating, and diarrhea.
- Reduced edema or ascites.
- Decreased urine output.
- Alleviated symptoms of depression and lowered consciousness, thus reducing pain and other distressing symptoms [181].

#### 7.1.4.3 Family Support during near to Death

It is imperative that the family possesses comprehensive information regarding the appropriate channels to contact upon the demise of a child, along with guidelines for immediate action and protocols for postponement of certain tasks. Furthermore, the ability to engage in discussions concerning their preferences regarding post-death matters, including funeral preparations, is of significant importance.

#### 7.1.4.4 Bereavement Support Care

- Offer empathy and support.
- Assist with procedural aspects.
- Deliver bereavement counseling to aid the family in managing their grief.
- Ensure the family experiences the belief that their child was cherished and looked after to the utmost [182].

### 7.1.5 Summary

The measures undertaken by healthcare professionals approaching the end-of-life care to child can significantly influence the quality of their passing. This, in turn, may facilitate parental coping mechanisms following the child's demise or engender considerable grief. The cornerstone of effective care management lies in professional evaluation, strategic planning, clear communication, and the provision of sufficient resources. It is imperative that all members of the healthcare team enhance their proficiency in relevant areas, including symptom control, nursing care, and comprehension of the family's religious and spiritual needs.

## 7.2 Pediatric Advance Care Planning

### 7.2.1 Introduction

The advancements in technology within the medical domain have had a substantial impact on enhancing survival rates and elevating the quality of life for children across different age groups who are battling chronic, life-limiting ailments. The procedure of advance care planning entails considerations of life-sustaining interventions and the establishment of long-term care goals. The ethical commitment of pediatric healthcare professionals to acquiring expertise in this specific area of medical care is of paramount importance. The purpose of this statement is to offer healthcare professionals guidance on how to engage in advance care planning discussions with pediatric patients in diverse healthcare environments [62].

### 7.2.2 Advance Care Planning

Advance care planning is an essential component of conventional dialogues concerning treatment plans, with a primary emphasis on curative measures and the provision of care rather than its exclusion. It incorporates a comprehensive spectrum of healthcare goals and treatments, spanning both immediate and long-term perspectives. This could entail the development of official advance medical directives, which outline the specific medical interventions that will be administered or withheld from the patient.

Proficient advance care planning provides multifaceted benefits, encompassing both procedural and substantive advantages. On a procedural basis, it promotes enhanced two-way communication, whereas on a substantive basis, it guarantees the explicit articulation of the patient's care plan. Through the effective implementation of advance care planning, healthcare professionals have the ability to maintain consistency between care objectives and the predetermined treatment plan, regardless of whether the focus is on cure or palliative care.

Even in the final stages, children with life-threatening conditions can receive interventions like intubation that are considered necessary to maintain life. It is crucial, prior to the occurrence of a life-threatening event, to deliberate on the necessity of initiating such interventions. Early discussions between parents and children help them make decisions that are consistent with their own values and care goals. This evaluation process must assess the likelihood of achieving the desired outcomes with the proposed interventions, including intubation, chest compressions, and defibrillation [183, 184].

#### 7.2.2.1 Elements of Pediatric Advance Care Planning

- Foster a collaborative partnership with the family.
- Participate in discussions regarding the prognosis and expected future outcomes.
- Consider the values pertaining to quality of life held by both the patient and their family, acknowledging the subjective nature of defining a "normal" quality of life.
- Assess the objectives, worries, and overall strengths, values, and needs of the patient and their family.
- Gain insight into the family's perspectives on the qualities of an ideal parent.
- It is important to effectively convey the potential advantages and disadvantages of treatment alternatives, taking into account their consequences in consultation with the patient and their family.
- Provide treatment recommendations, including strategies for responding in case treatments become burdensome or the patient's condition deteriorates.
- Explore the preferences of the child and family concerning end-of-life care, encompassing strategies for symptom management, resuscitation efforts, and the preferred place of death [185].

#### 7.2.2.2 The Significance of the Multidisciplinary Team in Advance Care Planning

- Advance care planning is a vital element of the expected standard of care for pediatricians and healthcare professionals dedicated to treating children with chronic, life-threatening illnesses.
- As healthcare professionals, it is our responsibility to initiate these crucial discussions instead of waiting for patient and family inquiries.
- These discussions should initiate promptly and sustain consistently throughout the treat-

ment process, preferably prior to any critical circumstances and as the care objectives are further developed or modified.

- It is crucial to elucidate and record the patient's preferences regarding emergency and life-sustaining treatments, including cardiopulmonary resuscitation (CPR), in order to ensure proper communication of these directives to other healthcare professionals, such as home caregivers and school educators [186].
- The inclusion of palliative care in the healthcare strategy for children suffering from serious illnesses that negatively impact their quality of life should be taken into account when discussing treatment goals, if applicable.
- Specialists in pediatric palliative care should be engaged from the outset of discussions regarding treatment goals. Prior to the child being at imminent risk of dying, it is advisable to initiate discussions regarding palliative care.
- It is imperative that pediatric healthcare professionals advocate for the standardization of legislation across various jurisdictions pertaining to advance directives for minors. Additionally, there exists a significant opportunity to undertake research on the subject of advance care planning among minors facing life-threatening conditions [187, 188].

#### 7.2.2.3 Implementation Strategies for Facilitating Advance Care Planning (ACP)

1. **Initiate Early Discussions on Treatment Goals and Options for ACP.** Engage in conversations about treatment objectives and potential options for advance care planning (ACP) at the outset. Ensure ongoing dialogue throughout the progression of a medical illness to refine and adjust the advance care plan as necessary.
2. **Organize Family Discussions on Advance Care Planning for Older Minors:** Encourage the facilitation or recommendation of family conversation focused on advance care planning for older minors identified with significant health conditions. Promote a transparent discussion among family members to ensure their comprehension and participation in the decision-making framework.
3. **Collaborate with a Multidisciplinary Team:** Start discussing with a varied group of healthcare providers, including pediatricians, family physicians, specialists in specific areas, nurses, social workers, spiritual advisors, educators, and others [189].

### 7.2.3 Summary

Advance care planning constitutes a crucial component of the healthcare services for individuals with life-limiting conditions, encompassing both pediatric and adult populations. Healthcare practitioners are advised to undergo comprehensive education to ensure they possess the confidence required to initiate conversations regarding these matters with children and their families. It is of paramount importance for them to familiarize themselves with the available resources in both hospital and community environments that can be utilized to deliver a comprehensive, family-centered approach designed to facilitate the implementation of advance care plans for these children. Furthermore, significant efforts are required, concentrating on policy and legislation, to address the current gaps related to the formalization of advance directives for minors.

## 7.3 Compassion Fatigue in Pediatric Palliative Care Professionals

### 7.3.1 Introduction

In the realm of healthcare, the process of facing the demise of a child is significantly more distressing and traumatic compared to the loss of an adult. Compassion fatigue, burnout, and satisfaction in compassion are critical elements that can have detrimental effects on the personal well-being and job performance of healthcare professionals (Fig. 7.1). Compassion fatigue (CF) represents the distress faced by caregivers due to

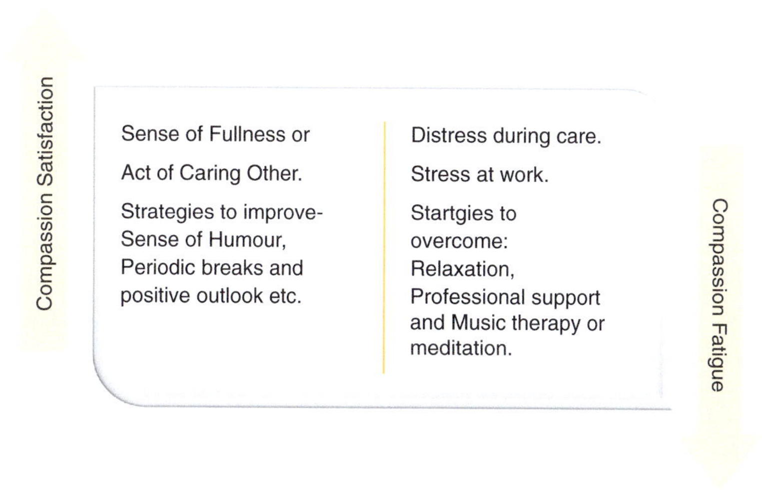


**Fig. 7.1** Diagrammatic representation of compassion satisfaction and compassion fatigue. This figure is researcher-made design and has not been adapted from any resource

continuous interaction with patients who are in pain. On the other hand, burnout (BO) is defined as occupational stress that is the consequence of a discrepancy between the demands of the job and the resources that are at the caregiver's disposal [190, 191].

Compassion fatigue represents a significant risk for professionals engaged in supporting individuals experiencing trauma. It is imperative to acknowledge that, even within a well-functioning team committed to adopting empathetic and supportive strategies with bereaved families following a child's death, it is inevitable for all team members to at some point encounter the adverse effects that accompany such compassionate involvement [192].

#### 7.3.1.1 Implementing Measures to Mitigate Compassion Fatigue

- Implemented measures encompass the establishment of professional boundaries, seeking support from colleagues and supervisors through reflection, engaging in physical exercise, and participating in non-work-related social activities.
- The interventions include cognitive training, educational programs, relaxation techniques, and a six-week meditation program administered via smartphone applications. Furthermore, music therapy is utilized as an additional intervention.
- The elements of well-being that are addressed encompass the search for spiritual significance, receiving assistance, and employing a blend of problem-focused and emotion-focused coping strategies.
- In addition, the program incorporates self-care strategies such as participating in palliative care training, developing effective communication skills, and nurturing personal hobbies [193–196].
- An educational program, based on simulation, is created to help reduce anxiety among graduate nurses working in end-of-life care [197].
- The need to enhance infrastructure, including ensuring adequate equipment and facilities, is imperative. Additionally, the recruitment and retention of an ample workforce is crucial. Equitable and fair compensation for palliative care professionals is of significant importance. Furthermore, workload can be alleviated by establishing restrictions on the allocation of patients to each caregiver [198].

#### 7.3.1.2 Compassion Satisfaction

Compassion satisfaction pertains to the individual and organizational fulfillment experienced as a result of engaging in challenging yet rewarding endeavors of delivering empathetic care to individuals facing crises. It encompasses the joy derived from assisting others and the conviction that one's professional contributions hold significance and value. Individuals engaged in palliative care may perceive diverse levels of satisfaction or gratification in their respective roles. The concept of compassion satisfaction pertains to the emotional contentment derived from the act of supporting others.

#### 7.3.1.3 Strategies to Improve Compassion Satisfaction

- A great sense of humor.
- Positive cognitive outlooks.
- Periodic breaks from professional responsibilities can also contribute to the relaxation process for individuals. These elements, in turn, contribute to the enhanced satisfaction levels frequently reported among pediatric care professionals [192, 199].

### 7.3.2 Summary

The phenomenon of compassion fatigue is a foreseeable and prevalent reaction to the routine duty of caring for terminally ill children. The symptoms of compassion fatigue frequently resemble those observed in trauma responses. This condition has the capacity to induce personal distress among healthcare professionals and to complicate the interactions between these professionals and the children and families under their care.

# References


1. Saunders C. The management of patients in the terminal stage. Cancer. 1960;6:403–17.
2. Abbasi P, Yoosefi Lebni J, Nouri P, Ziapour A, Jalali A. The obstacles to organ donation following brain death in Iran: a qualitative study. BMC Med Ethics. 2020;21(1):1–9.
3. Hanks GW. Oxford textbook of palliative medicine. USA: Oxford University Press; 2011.
4. Organization WH. Integrating palliative care and symptom relief into paediatrics: a WHO guide for health-care planners, implementers and managers. 2018.
5. Downing J. Children's palliative care: an international case-based manual. London: Springer; 2020.
6. Connor S, Morris C, Jaramillo E, Harding R, Cleary J, Haste B, et al. Global atlas of palliative care. London: Worldwide Hospice and Palliative Care Alliance; 2020. Report No.: 978-0-9928277-2-4.
7. Ghanbari Motlagh ATM. Theoretical foundations and comparative studies in supportive and palliative care system Cancer. Tehran: Ministry of Health, Treatment and Medical Education; 2018.
8. F. HM. Designing and implementing a hospital-based palliative care system: a participatory action research approach. Tehran: Islamic Azad University of Medical Sciences; 2020.
9. Jabbari A, Sohrabi K, Niaraees Zavare AS. Hospital-based palliative care models: advantages and limitations. Journal of Health Administration. 2021;24(2):45–58. https://doi.org/10.52547/jha.24.2.45.
10. Ghanbari Motlagh A, Tahmasebi M. Theoretical foundations and comparative studies in supportive and palliative care system Cancer. Tehran: Ministry of Health, Treatment and Medical Education; 2018 Jan.
11. Castro MCF, Fuly PSC, Santos MLSC, Chagas MC. Total pain and comfort theory: implications in the care to patients in oncology palliative care. Rev Gaucha Enferm. 2021;42:e20200311.
12. Homani MF. Designing and implementing a hospital-based palliative care system: a participatory action research approach [PhD thesis]. Tehran: Tehran Islamic Azad University of Medical Sciences; 2020.
13. Wiencek C, Coyne P. Palliative care delivery models. Seminars in oncology nursing. Elsevier; 2014.
14. Word Health Organization (WHO). Planning and implementing palliative care services: a guide for programme managers. Geneva: World Health Organization; 2016. Report No.: 9789241565417.
15. Pantilat SZ, Rabow MW, Kerr KM, Markowitz AJ. Palliative Care in California: the business case for hospital-based programs. California: California heathcare foundation; 2007. Report No.: 1-933795-25-5.
16. Basol N. The integration of palliative care into the emergency department. Turkish. J Emerg Med. 2015;15(2):100–7. https://doi.org/10.5505/1304.7361.2015.65983.
17. Mercadante S, Gregoretti C, Cortegiani A. Palliative care in intensive care units: why, where, what, who, when, how. BMC Anesthesiol. 2018;18(1):1–6. https://doi.org/10.1186/s12871-018-0574-9.
18. El-Jawahri A, Greer JA, Temel JS. Does palliative care improve outcomes for patients with incurable illness? A review of the evidence. J Support Oncol. 2011;9(3):87–94. https://doi.org/10.1016/j.suponc.2011.03.003.
19. Brock KE, Snaman JM, Kaye EC, Bower KA, Weaver MS, Baker JN, et al. Models of pediatric palliative oncology outpatient care—benefits, challenges, and opportunities. J Oncol Pract. 2019;15(9):476–87. https://doi.org/10.1200/JOP.19.00100.
20. Kaye EC, Friebert S, Baker JN. Early integration of palliative care for children with high-risk cancer and their families. Pediatr Blood Cancer. 2016;63(4):593–7. https://doi.org/10.1002/pbc.25848.
21. Salins N, Hughes S, Preston N. Palliative care in paediatric oncology: an update. Curr Oncol Rep. 2022;24(2):175–86. https://doi.org/10.1007/s11912-021-01170-3.
22. Khanali ML. Designing palliative Care model in children with cancer [PhD thesis]. Tehran: Shahid Beheshti University of Medical Sciences; 2018.



N. Javadi-Pashaki et al., *Interdisciplinary Pediatric Palliative Care*,
https://doi.org/10.1007/978-981-97-9587-1

23. Wolfe J, Hinds P, Sourkes B. Textbook of interdisciplinary pediatric palliative Care: expert consult. Premium ed. Philadelphia: Elsevier Health Sciences; 2011.
24. Hays RM, Valentine J, Haynes G, Geyer JR, Villareale N, Mckinstry B, et al. The Seattle Pediatric Palliative Care Project: effects on family satisfaction and health-related quality of life. J Palliat Med. 2006;9(3):716–28. https://doi.org/10.1089/jpm.2006.9.716.
25. Klassen AF, Raina P, McIntosh C, Sung L, Klaassen RJ, O'Donnell M, et al. Parents of children with cancer: which factors explain differences in health-related quality of life. Int J Cancer. 2011;129(5):1190–8. https://doi.org/10.1002/ijc.25737.
26. Docherty SL, Thaxton C, Allison C, Barfield RC, Tamburro RF. The nursing dimension of providing palliative care to children and adolescents with cancer. Clin Med Insights Pediatr. 2012;6:CMPed. S8208. https://doi.org/10.4137/CMPed.S8208.
27. Word Health Organization (WHO). Integrating palliative care and symptom relief into paediatrics: a WHO guide for health-care planners, implementers and managers. Geneva: World Health Organization; 2018. Report No.: 978-92-4-151445-3.
28. Caruso Brown AE, Howard SC, Baker JN, Ribeiro RC, Lam CG. Reported availability and gaps of pediatric palliative care in low- and middle-income countries: a systematic review of published data. J Palliat Med. 2014;17(12):1369–83. https://doi.org/10.1089/jpm.2014.0095.
29. Kwame A, Petrucka PM. Communication in nurse-patient interaction in healthcare settings in sub-Saharan Africa: a scoping review. Int J Afr Nurs Sci. 2020;12:100198.
30. Goldman A, Hain R, Liben S. Oxford textbook of palliative care for children. Oxford Textbooks in Palliative; 2012.
31. Norouzinia R, Aghabarari M, Shiri M, Karimi M, Samami E. Communication barriers perceived by nurses and patients. Global J Health Sci. 2016;8(6):65.
32. Fortinash KM, Worret PAH. Psychiatric mental health nursing. Elsevier Health Sciences; 2011.
33. Reynolds W. The measurement and development of empathy in nursing. Routledge; 2017.
34. Dryden P, Greenshields S. Communicating with children and young people. Br J Nurs. 2020;29(20):1164–6.
35. Winnicott C, Kanter J. Communicating with children. 1997.
36. Kaye P. Breaking bad news: a ten step approach. Scion Publishing Ltd; 2023.
37. Buckman RA. Breaking bad news: the SPIKES strategy. Commun Oncol. 2005;2(2):138–42.
38. Ptacek JT, Eberhardt TL. Breaking bad news: a review of the literature. JAMA. 1996;276(6):496–502.
39. Vandekieft GK. Breaking bad news. Am Fam Physician. 2001;64(12):1975–9.
40. Nunn K. Delivering bad news. J Paediatr Child Health. 2019;55(6):617–20.
41. Ebrahimi A. Communication and communication skills. Tehran: Tehran University of Medical Sciences; 2011.
42. Sutar R, Chaudhary P, Yadav V. Prevalence of collusion in cancer communications: a meta-analysis. Psycho-Oncology. 2022;31(3):372–87.
43. Deffenbacher JL. Ideal treatment package for adults with anger disorders. Anger disorders. Taylor & Francis; 2014. p. 151–72.
44. Faupel A. Dealing with anger and aggression. Working with emotions. Routledge; 2003. p. 113–26.
45. Weiss RS. The nature and causes of grief. In: Stroebe MS, Hansson RO, Schut H, Stroebe W, editors. Handbook of bereavement research and practice: advances in theory and intervention. American Psychological Association; 2008. p. 29–44.
46. Hunt J, Talawadekar P, Friedel M. Anticipatory grief and bereavement support. In: Children's palliative care: an international case-based manual. Springer Cham; 2020. p. 201–10.
47. Morris K. Bereavement in children and young people. Grief, loss and bereavement. Routledge; 2013. p. 35–51.
48. Lancaster J. Developmental stages, grief, and a child's response to death. Pediatr Ann. 2011;40(5):277–81.
49. Open Resources for Nursing (Open RN), Ernstmeyer K, Christman E, editors. Nursing fundamentals [Internet]. Eau Claire (WI): Chippewa Valley Technical College; 2021. Chapter 17 grief and loss. https://www.ncbi.nlm.nih.gov/books/NBK591827/.
50. Lowey SE. Nursing care at the end of life: what every clinician should know. Open SUNY Textbooks; 2015.
51. Kübler-Ross E. On death and dying. New York: Routledge; 1969/2009.
52. American Nurses Association. Nursing informatics: scope and standards of practice. 2015.
53. Oates JR, Maani CV. Death and dying. 2019.
54. O'Connor J. Children and grief: helping your child understand death. Revell; 2004.
55. Finkbeiner AK. After the death of a child: living with the loss through the years. Simon and Schuster; 2012.
56. Claire E. Spirituality. In: Kimberly Ernstmeyer EC, editor. Nursing fundamentals. Chippewa Valley Technical College; 2021.
57. Word Health Organization (WHO). WHO definition of palliative care. https://www.who.int/cancer/palliative/definition/en/index.html. 2002.
58. Hyman C, Handal PJ. Definitions and evaluation of religion and spirituality items by religious professionals: a pilot study. J Relig Health. 2006;45:264–82.
59. Taves A. Religious experience reconsidered: a building-block approach to the study of religion

and other special things. Princeton University Press; 2009.
60. Puchalski CM, Vitillo R, Hull SK, Reller N. Improving the spiritual dimension of whole person care: reaching national and international consensus. J Palliat Med. 2014;17(6):642–56.
61. Ferrell BR, Twaddle ML, Melnick A, Meier DE. National Consensus Project Clinical Practice Guidelines for Quality Palliative Care Guidelines, 4th Edition. J Palliat Med. 2018;21(12):1684–9.
62. Himelstein BP, Hilden JM, Boldt AM, Weissman D. Pediatric palliative care. N Engl J Med. 2004;350(17):1752–62.
63. Nissen RD, Viftrup DT, Hvidt NC. The process of spiritual care. Front Psychol. 2021;12:674453.
64. Fernando G, Hughes S. Team approaches in palliative care: a review of the literature. Int J Palliat Nurs. 2019;25(9):444–51.
65. Speck P. Team or group–spot the difference. In: Teamwork in palliative care: fulfilling or frustrating. Oxford University Press; 2006. p. 7–23.
66. Papadatou D, Bluebond-Langner M, Goldman A, Wolfe J, Hinds P, Sourkes B. The team. In: Textbook of interdisciplinary pediatric palliative care. Philadelphia: Elsevier/Saunders; 2011. p. 55–63.
67. Papadatou D. In the face of death: professionals who care for the dying and the bereaved. Springer Publishing Company; 2009.
68. Pasinski D. The Helper's Journey: Working with People Facing Grief, Loss, and Life-Threatening Illness. By Dale Larson: Champaign, IL: Research Press, 1993. 279 pp. $11.95 softbound. Taylor & Francis; 1997.
69. Steele F. The open organization: the impact of secrecy and disclosure on people and organizations. (No Title). 1975.
70. Senge PM. The fifth discipline: the art and practice of the learning organization. Broadway Business; 2006.
71. Crawford GB, Price SD. Team working: palliative care as a model of interdisciplinary practice. Med J Aust. 2003;179(6):S32.
72. Ramirez A, Addington-Hall J, Richards M. ABC of palliative care: the carers. BMJ. 1998;316(7126):208–11.
73. Kirby E, Broom A, Good P. The role and significance of nurses in managing transitions to palliative care: a qualitative study. BMJ Open. 2014;4(9):e006026.
74. Puchalski CM. Spirituality and end-of-life care: a time for listening and caring. J Palliat Med. 2002;5(2):289–94.
75. Øvretveit J. Five ways to describe a multidisciplinary team. J Interprof Care. 1996;10(2):163–71.
76. Mullick A, Martin J, Sallnow L. An introduction to advance care planning in practice. BMJ. 2013;347:f6064.
77. Morris S, Wilmot A, Hill M, Ockenden N, Payne S. A narrative literature review of the contribution of volunteers in end-of-life care services. Palliat Med. 2013;27(5):428–36.
78. Kumar SK. Kerala, India: a regional community-based palliative care model. J Pain Symptom Manag. 2007;33(5):623–7.
79. Twomey C, Byrne M, Leahy T. Steps towards effective teamworking in community mental health teams. Ir J Psychol Med. 2014;31(1):51–9.
80. Feiger SM, Schmitt MH. Collegiality in interdisciplinary health teams: its measurement and its effects. Soc Sci Med (1967). 1979;13:217–29.
81. Mahmood-Yousuf K, Munday D, King N, Dale J. Interprofessional relationships and communication in primary palliative care: impact of the Gold Standards Framework. Br J Gen Pract. 2008;58(549):256–63.
82. Klarare A, Hagelin CL, Fürst CJ, Fossum B. Team interactions in specialized palliative care teams: a qualitative study. J Palliat Med. 2013;16(9):1062–9.
83. Liebig B, Piccini C. Inter-professional communication in palliative care: general practitioners and specialists in Switzerland. Clin Case Report Rev. 2017;3(2):1–5.
84. Faulkner A. ABC of palliative care: communication with patients, families, and other professionals. BMJ. 1998;316(7125):130–2.
85. Kurer M, Zekri J. Breaking bad news: can we get it right? Libyan J Med. 2008;3(4):200–3.
86. Oliver DP, Peck M. Inside the interdisciplinary team experiences of hospice social workers. J Soc Work End Life Palliat Care. 2006;2(3):7–21.
87. Huang S-T, Good M, Zauszniewski JA. The effectiveness of music in relieving pain in cancer patients: a randomized controlled trial. Int J Nurs Stud. 2010;47(11):1354–62.
88. Silbermann M, Pitsillides B, Al-Alfi N, Omran S, Al-Jabri K, Elshamy K, et al. Multidisciplinary care team for cancer patients and its implementation in several Middle Eastern countries. Ann Oncol. 2013;24:vii41–vii7.
89. Bélanger E, Rodríguez C, Groleau D, Légaré F, MacDonald ME, Marchand R. Patient participation in palliative care decisions: an ethnographic discourse analysis. Int J Qual Stud Health Well Being. 2016;11(1):32438.
90. Baldacchino D. Spiritual care education of health care professionals. MDPI; 2015.
91. Green S. Making it right in the end: conflict on the hospice interdisciplinary team. 2017. Social Work Master's Clinical Research Papers, 741.
92. Kamal AH, Bull JH, Wolf SP, Swetz KM, Shanafelt TD, Ast K, et al. Prevalence and predictors of burnout among hospice and palliative care clinicians in the US. J Pain Symptom Manag. 2020;59(5): e6–e13.
93. Kaës R. Réalité psychique et souffrance dans les institutions. L'institution et les institutions. 1987:1–46.

94. Sourkes BM. Armfuls of time: the psychological experience of the child with a life-threatening. illness: Routledge; 2008.
95. Bluebond-Langner M. In the shadow of illness: parents and siblings of the chronically ill child. Princeton University Press; 2000.
96. Bluebond-Langner M, Belasco JB, Goldman A, Belasco C. Understanding parents' approaches to care and treatment of children with cancer when standard therapy has failed. J Clin Oncol. 2007;25(17):2414–9.
97. Payne M, Campling J. Teamwork in multiprofessional care. Springer; 2000.
98. Wolfe J, Klar N, Grier HE, Duncan J, Salem-Schatz S, Emanuel EJ, et al. Understanding of prognosis among parents of children who died of cancer: impact on treatment goals and integration of palliative care. JAMA. 2000;284(19):2469–75.
99. Foster TL. Pediatric palliative care revisited: a vision to add life. J Hosp Palliat Nurs. 2007;9(4):212–9.
100. Monterosso L, Kristjanson LJ. Supportive and palliative care needs of families of children who die from cancer: an Australian study. Palliat Med. 2008;22(1):59–69.
101. Papadatou D, Papazoglou I, Petraki D, Bellali T. Mutual support among nurses who provide care to dying children. Illn Crisis Loss. 1999;7(1):37–48.
102. Vachon M. Recent research into staff stress in palliative care. Eur J Palliat Care. 1997;4:99–104.
103. Winnicott DW. The maturational processes and the facilitating environment: studies in the theory of emotional development. Routledge; 2018.
104. Kahn WA. Holding fast: the struggle to create resilient caregiving organizations. Routledge; 2004.
105. Kahn WA. Holding environments at work. J Appl Behav Sci. 2001;37(3):260–79.
106. Ketchum LT, Trist E. All teams are not equal. London: Sage; 1992.
107. Browning DM, Solomon MZ, Team IfPPCI. The initiative for pediatric palliative care: an interdisciplinary educational approach for healthcare professionals. J Pediatr Nurs. 2005;20(5):326–34.
108. Liben S, Papadatou D, Wolfe J. Paediatric palliative care: challenges and emerging ideas. Lancet. 2008;371(9615):852–64.
109. Wolfe J, Grier HE, Klar N, Levin SB, Ellenbogen JM, Salem-Schatz S, et al. Symptoms and suffering at the end of life in children with cancer. N Engl J Med. 2000;342(5):326–33.
110. Gade G, Venohr I, Conner D, McGrady K, Beane J, Richardson RH, et al. Impact of an inpatient palliative care team: a randomized controlled trial. J Palliat Med. 2008;11(2):180–90.
111. Drake R, Frost J, Collins JJ. The symptoms of dying children. J Pain Symptom Manag. 2003;26(1):594–603.
112. Gulve A. Pain assessment. In: Pain management: From basics to clinical practice. Churchill Livingstone; 2008. p. 213.
113. Reynolds LA, Tansey E. Innovation in pain management: the Wellcome Trust Centre for the History of Medicine at UCL; 2004.
114. Timm H. Transformation of the concepts and practice of total pain and total care: 30 years of Danish hospices. Front Sociol. 2023;8:1145131.
115. Portenoy RK, Payne D, Jacobsen P. Breakthrough pain: characteristics and impact in patients with cancer pain. Pain. 1999;81(1–2):129–34.
116. Hockenberry MJ, Wilson D. Wong's Nursing Care of Infants and Children-E-Book: Wong's Nursing Care of Infants and Children-E-Book. Elsevier Health Sciences; 2018.
117. Hartrick CT, Kovan JP, Shapiro S. The numeric rating scale for clinical pain measurement: a ratio measure? Pain Pract. 2003;3(4):310–6.
118. Krechel SW, Bildner J. CRIES: a new neonatal postoperative pain measurement score. Initial testing of validity and reliability. Pediatr Anesth. 1995;5(1):53–61.
119. McGrath P, Johnson G, Goodman J, Schillinger J. The development and validation of a behavioral pain scale for children: the children's hospital of eastern Ontario pain scale (CHEOPS). Pain. 1984;18:S24.
120. Stevens BJ, Gibbins S, Yamada J, Dionne K, Lee G, Johnston C, et al. The premature infant pain profile-revised (PIPP-R): initial validation and feasibility. Clin J Pain. 2014;30(3):238–43.
121. Organization WH. Persisting pain in children package: WHO guidelines on the pharmacological treatment of persisting pain in children with medical illnesses. 2012.
122. Ventafridda V, Saita L, Ripamonti C, De Conno F. WHO guidelines for the use of analgesics in cancer pain. Int J Tissue React. 1985;7(1):93–6.
123. Orhan ME, Bilgin F, Ergin A, Dere K, Güzeldemir ME. Pain treatment practice according to the WHO analgesic ladder in cancer patients: eight years experience of a single center. Agri. 2008;20(4):38–44.
124. Arafa SK, Elsayed AA, Hagras AM, Shama AAA. Pediatric postoperative pain control with quadratus lumborum block and dexamethasone in two routes with bupivacaine: a prospective randomized controlled clinical trial. Pain Physician. 2022;25(7):E987–98.
125. Lence T, Thinnes R, Foster AJ, Cooper CS, Lockwood GM, Ten Eyck P, et al. Opioids and pediatric urology: a prospective study evaluating prescribing habits and patient postoperative pain and narcotic utilization. J Pediatr Urol. 2023;19(3):295.e1–8.
126. Di Sarno L, Gatto A, Korn D, Pansini V, Curatola A, Ferretti S, et al. Pain management in pediatric age. An update. Acta Biomed. 2023;94(4):e2023174.
127. Agrawal US, Sarin J, Bakhshi S, Garg R. Challenges and opportunities in providing palliative care services to children with a life-limiting illness: a systematic review. Natl Med J India. 2022;35(5):284.

128. Ismail A. The challenges of providing effective pain management for children in the pediatric intensive care unit. Pain Manag Nurs. 2016;17(6):372–83.
129. Sahiner NC, Bal MD. The effects of three different distraction methods on pain and anxiety in children. J Child Health Care. 2016;20(3):277–85.
130. Short S, Pace G, Birnbaum C. Nonpharmacologic techniques to assist in pediatric pain management. Clin Pediatr Emerg Med. 2017;18(4):256–60.
131. Vagnoli L, Bettini A, Amore E, De Masi S, Messeri A. Relaxation-guided imagery reduces perioperative anxiety and pain in children: a randomized study. Eur J Pediatr. 2019;178:913–21.
132. Yasaman Yaghobi SP, Panahi L, Haryahchi K. Pain management and acupressure. Salehian: Tehran; 2018.
133. Friedrichsdorf SJ, Goubert L. Pediatric pain treatment and prevention for hospitalized children. Pain Report. 2020;5(1):e804.
134. Hauch H, Kriwy P, Hahn A, Dettmeyer R, Zimmer K-P, Neubauer B, et al. Gastrointestinal symptoms in children with life-limiting conditions receiving palliative home care. Front Pediatr. 2021;9: 654531.
135. Jalmsell L, Kreicbergs U, Onelöv E, Steineck G, Henter J-I. Symptoms affecting children with malignancies during the last month of life: a nationwide follow-up. Pediatrics. 2006;117(4):1314–20.
136. Baines MJ. ABC of palliative care. Nausea, vomiting, and intestinal obstruction. BMJ. Br Med J. 1997;315(7116):1148.
137. Mancini I, Bruera E. Constipation in advanced cancer patients. Support Care Cancer. 1998;6(4):356–64.
138. Santucci G, Mack JW. Common gastrointestinal symptoms in pediatric palliative care: nausea, vomiting, constipation, anorexia, cachexia. Pediatr Clin N Am. 2007;54(5):673–89.
139. Fallon M, O'Neill B. ABC of palliative care: constipation and diarrhoea. BMJ. 1997;315(7118):1293–6.
140. Ladas EJ, Post-White J, Hawks R, Taromina K. Evidence for symptom management in the child with cancer. J Pediatr Hematol Oncol. 2006;28(9):601–15.
141. Ladas EJ, Sacks N, Meacham L, Henry D, Enriquez L, Lowry G, et al. A multidisciplinary review of nutrition considerations in the pediatric oncology population: a perspective from children's oncology group. Nutr Clin Pract. 2005;20(4):377–93.
142. Bruera E. ABC of palliative care: anorexia, cachexia, and nutrition. BMJ. 1997;315(7117):1219–22.
143. McKinlay A. Nutritional support in patients with advanced cancer: permission to fall out? Proc Nutr Soc. 2004;63(3):431–5.
144. Buijs EA, Reiss IK, Kraemer U, Andrinopoulou E-R, Zwiers AJ, Ince C, et al. Increasing mean arterial blood pressure and heart rate with catecholaminergic drugs does not improve the microcirculation in children with congenital diaphragmatic hernia: a prospective cohort study. Pediatr Crit Care Med. 2014;15(4):343–54.
145. Carter BS, Howenstein M, Gilmer MJ, Throop P, France D, Whitlock JA. Circumstances surrounding the deaths of hospitalized children: opportunities for pediatric palliative care. Pediatrics. 2004;114(3):e361–e6.
146. Jennings A, Davies A, Higgins J, Gibbs J, Broadley K. A systematic review of the use of opioids in the management of dyspnoea. Thorax. 2002;57(11):939–44.
147. Craig F, Henderson EM, Bluebond-Langner M. Management of respiratory symptoms in paediatric palliative care. Curr Opin Support Palliat Care. 2015;9(3):217–26.
148. Batra PS, Holinger LD. Etiology and management of pediatric hemoptysis. Arch Otolaryngol Head Neck Surg. 2001;127(4):377–82.
149. Tom LW, Weisman RA, Handler SD. Hemoptysis in children. Ann Otol Rhinol Laryngol. 1980;89(5):419–24.
150. Bennett DS. Depression among children with chronic medical problems: a meta-analysis. J Pediatr Psychol. 1994;19(2):149–69.
151. Feudtner C, Kang TI, Hexem KR, Friedrichsdorf SJ, Osenga K, Siden H, et al. Pediatric palliative care patients: a prospective multicenter cohort study. Pediatrics. 2011;127(6):1094–101.
152. Varni JW, Seid M, Kurtin PS. PedsQL™ 4.0: Reliability and validity of the Pediatric Quality of Life Inventory™ Version 4.0 Generic Core Scales in healthy and patient populations. Med Care. 2001;39(8):800–12.
153. Irwin DE, Gross HE, Stucky BD, Thissen D, DeWitt EM, Lai JS, et al. Development of six PROMIS pediatrics proxy-report item banks. Health Qual Life Outcomes. 2012;10:1–13.
154. Muris P, Merckelbach H, Ollendick T, King N, Bogie N. Three traditional and three new childhood anxiety questionnaires: their reliability and validity in a normal adolescent sample. Behav Res Ther. 2002;40(7):753–72.
155. Pilkonis PA, Choi SW, Reise SP, Stover AM, Riley WT, Cella D, et al. Item banks for measuring emotional distress from the Patient-Reported Outcomes Measurement Information System (PROMIS®): depression, anxiety, and anger. Assessment. 2011;18(3):263–83.
156. Collins JJ, Devine TD, Dick GS, Johnson EA, Kilham HA, Pinkerton CR, et al. The measurement of symptoms in young children with cancer: the validation of the Memorial Symptom Assessment Scale in children aged 7–12. J Pain Symptom Manag. 2002;23(1):10–6.
157. Chan A, Woodruff RK. Communicating with patients with advanced cancer. J Palliat Care. 1997;13(3):29–33.
158. Rasmussen LA, Grégoire M-C. Challenging neurological symptoms in paediatric palliative care: an approach to symptom evaluation and management in children with neurological impairment. Paediatr Child Health. 2015;20(3):159–65.

159. Mody K, Kaur S, Mauer EA, Gerber LM, Greenwald BM, Silver G, et al. Benzodiazepines and development of delirium in critically ill children: estimating the causal effect. Crit Care Med. 2018;46(9):1486–91.
160. Falsaperla R, Marino S, Moscheo C, Tardino LG, Marino SD, Sciuto C, et al. Need for palliative care from birth to infancy in pediatric patients with neurological diseases. Clin Exp Pediatr. 2023; 66(8):350.
161. Wusthoff CJ, Shellhaas RA, Licht DJ. Management of common neurologic symptoms in pediatric palliative care: seizures, agitation, and spasticity. Pediatr Clin N Am. 2007;54(5):709–33.
162. Pace A, Villani V, Di Lorenzo C, Guariglia L, Maschio M, Pompili A, et al. Epilepsy in the end-of-life phase in patients with high-grade gliomas. J Neuro-Oncol. 2013;111:83–6.
163. Kang S-Y, Um J-Y, Chung B-Y, Kim J-C, Park C-W, Kim H-O. Differential diagnosis and treatment of itching in children and adolescents. Biomedicines. 2021;9(8):919.
164. Yosipovitch G, Misery L, Proksch E, Metz M, Ständer S, Schmelz M. Skin barrier damage and itch: review of mechanisms, topical management and future directions. Acta Derm Venereol. 2019;99(13):1201.
165. Koumaki D, Kostakis G, Boumpoucheropoulos S, Ioannou P, Katoulis AC. A narrative review of management of wounds in palliative care setting. Ann Palliat Med. 2023;12(5):1089105–1105.
166. Ranade D, Collins N. Children with wounds: the importance of nutrition. HMP Communications, Malvern, PA; 2011. p. 14+.
167. Grocott P. Developing a tool for researching fungating wounds. World Wide Wounds. 2001;2001:15p.
168. West D. A palliative approach to the management of malodour from malignant fungating tumours. Int J Palliat Nurs. 2007;13(3):137–42.
169. Death CoA, Issues AKE-o-L. Dying in America: improving quality and honoring individual preferences near the end of life. 2015.
170. Ulrich CM, Mooney-Doyle K, Grady C. Communicating with pediatric families at end-of-life is not a fantasy. Am J Bioeth. 2018;18(1): 14–6.
171. Feudtner C. Collaborative communication in pediatric palliative care: a foundation for problem-solving and decision-making. Pediatr Clin N Am. 2007;54(5):583–607.
172. Blazin LJ, Cecchini C, Habashy C, Kaye EC, Baker JN. Communicating effectively in pediatric cancer care: translating evidence into practice. Children. 2018;5(3):40.
173. Santoro JD, Bennett M. Ethics of end of life decisions in pediatrics: a narrative review of the roles of caregivers, shared decision-making, and patient centered values. Behav Sci. 2018;8(5):42.
174. Muckaden M, Dighe M, Balaji P, Dhiliwal S, Tilve P, Jadhav S, et al. Paediatric palliative care: theory to practice. Indian J Palliat Care. 2011;17(Suppl):S52.
175. Ten Have H, Welie JV. Palliative sedation versus euthanasia: an ethical assessment. J Pain Symptom Manag. 2014;47(1):123–36.
176. Noyes M, Herbert A, Moloney S, Irving H, Bradford N. Location of end-of-life care of children with cancer: a systematic review of parent experiences. Pediatr Blood Cancer. 2022;69(6):e29621.
177. Collins JJ, Frager G. Pain and pain relief in pediatric end-of-life care. In: Bringing pain relief to children: treatment approaches. Totowa: Humana Press; 2006. p. 59–83.
178. Komatz K, Carter B. Pain and symptom management in pediatric palliative care. Pediatr Rev. 2015;36(12):527–34.
179. Carter BS, Jones PM. Evidence-based comfort care for neonates towards the end of life. In: Seminars in Fetal and Neonatal Medicine. Elsevier; 2013.
180. Billings JA. Comfort measures for the terminally Ill: is dehydration painful? Wiley Online Library; 1985. p. 808–10.
181. Sutcliffe J, Holmes S. Dehydration: burden or benefit to the dying patient? J Adv Nurs. 1994;19(1):71–6.
182. Currier JM, Neimeyer RA, Berman JS. The effectiveness of psychotherapeutic interventions for bereaved persons: a comprehensive quantitative review. Psychol Bull. 2008;134(5):648.
183. Linebarger JS, Johnson V, Boss RD. Guidance for pediatric end-of-life care. Pediatrics. 2022;149:5.
184. Mack JW, Wolfe J. Early integration of pediatric palliative care: for some children, palliative care starts at diagnosis. Curr Opin Pediatr. 2006;18(1):10–4.
185. Bennett HE, Duke S, Richardson A. Paediatric advance care planning in life-limiting conditions: scoping review of parent experiences. BMJ Support Palliat Care. 2023;13(2):161–73.
186. House SA, Schoo C, Ogilvie WA. Advance directives. StatPearls Publishing; 2017.
187. Lotz JD, Jox RJ, Borasio GD, Führer M. Pediatric advance care planning from the perspective of health care professionals: a qualitative interview study. Palliat Med. 2015;29(3):212–22.
188. Lusney N, van Breemen C, Lim E, Pawliuk C, Hussein Z. Pediatric advance care planning: a scoping review. Children. 2023;10(7):1179.
189. Tsai E, Society CP, Committee B. Advance care planning for paediatric patients. Paediatr Child Health. 2008;13(9):791–6.
190. Kase SM, Waldman ED, Weintraub AS. A cross-sectional pilot study of compassion fatigue, burnout, and compassion satisfaction in pediatric palliative care providers in the United States. Palliat Support Care. 2019;17(3):269–75.
191. Rourke MT. Compassion fatigue in pediatric palliative care providers. Pediatr Clin N Am. 2007;54(5):631–44.
192. Rico-Mena P, Güeita-Rodríguez J, Martino-Alba R, Castel-Sánchez M, Palacios-Ceña D. The emotional experience of caring for children in Pediatric Palliative Care: a qualitative study among a home-based Interdisciplinary Care Team. Children. 2023;10(4):700.

193. Baqeas MH, Davis J, Copnell B. Compassion fatigue and compassion satisfaction among palliative care health providers: a scoping review. BMC Palliat Care. 2021;20(1):88.
194. Hill RC, Dempster M, Donnelly M, McCorry NK. Improving the wellbeing of staff who work in palliative care settings: a systematic review of psychosocial interventions. Palliat Med. 2016;30(9):825–33.
195. Melvin CS. Professional compassion fatigue: what is the true cost of nurses caring for the dying? Int J Palliat Nurs. 2012;18(12):606–11.
196. Mota Vargas R, Mahtani-Chugani V, Solano Pallero M, Rivero Jiménez B, Cabo Domínguez R, Robles AV. The transformation process for palliative care professionals: the metamorphosis, a qualitative research study. Palliat Med. 2016;30(2):161–70.
197. Beavis J, Davis L, McKenzie S. Clinical supervision for support workers in paediatric palliative care: a literature review. Clin Child Psychol Psychiatry. 2021;26(1):191–206.
198. Popa MV, Mîndru DE, Hizanu M, Gurzu IL, Anton-Păduraru DT, Ştreangă V, et al., editors. Stress Factors for the Paediatric and Adult Palliative Care Multidisciplinary Team and Workplace Wellbeing Solutions. Healthcare; 2024. MDPI.
199. Stamm BH. Measuring compassion satisfaction as well as fatigue: developmental history of the compassion satisfaction and fatigue test. Treating compassion fatigue: Routledge; 2013. p. 107–19.

# Index




N. Javadi-Pashaki et al., *Interdisciplinary Pediatric Palliative Care*,
https://doi.org/10.1007/978-981-97-9587-1

MIX
Papier aus verantwortungsvollen Quellen
Paper from responsible sources
FSC® C105338

If you have any concerns about our products,
you can contact us on
**ProductSafety@springernature.com**

In case Publisher is established outside the EU,
the EU authorized representative is:
**Springer Nature Customer Service Center GmbH**
**Europaplatz 3, 69115 Heidelberg, Germany**

Printed by Libri Plureos GmbH
in Hamburg, Germany